# THE EVERYTHING

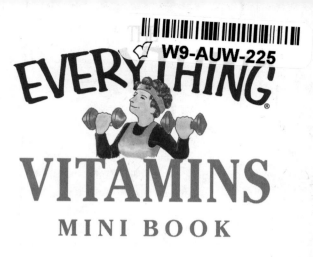

# VITAMINS

## MINI BOOK

Maureen Ternus, M.S., R.D.,
and Kitty Broihier, M.S., R.D.

Adams Media Corporation
Avon, Massachusetts

An Everything® Series Book.
"Everything" is a registered trademark of Adams Media Corporation.

Published by Adams Media Corporation
57 Littlefield Street, Avon, MA 02322
*www.adamsmedia.com*

ISBN: 1-58062-609-2

Printed in Canada.

J I H G F E D C B

Library of Congress Cataloging-in-Publication Data
available from the publisher.

This publication is designed to provide accurate and authoritative
information with regard to the subject matter covered. It is sold
with the understanding that the publisher is not engaged in ren-
dering legal, accounting, or other professional advice. If legal
advice or other expert assistance is required, the services of a
competent professional person should be sought.
— From a *Declaration of Principles* jointly adopted by a Committee of the
American Bar Association and a Committee of Publishers and Associations

Cover illustrations by Barry Littmann.
Interior illustrations by Barry Littmann.
Additional contributions by Susan Gaber.

*This book is available at quantity discounts for bulk purchases.
For information, call 1-800-872-5627.*

# Contents

# Introduction

Vitamin and mineral supplements make up the third-largest over-the-counter drug category in the United States and are among the most widely used nonprescription products today. According to recent reports, sales of these nutritional supplements increased by about $3.5 billion between 1994 and 1998, to nearly $5 billion.

These supplements are used by many in hopes of preventing the aging process and avoiding chronic diseases including cancer, heart disease, and diabetes. But are these "magic pills"

all they're cracked up to be? As public interest in
vitamin and mineral supplements has increased,
so has research on them. Once recommended
solely for the prevention and treatment of particular deficiency diseases, supplements are now
being studied for their potential health benefits.
A recent example is the recommendation to take
folic acid to prevent a certain type of birth
defect. The research was so compelling that the
U.S. Public Health Service now recommends that
all women of childbearing age consume 400
micrograms of folic acid per day via fortified
foods and/or supplements.

Still, there are a number of products
being sold today that may not be useful
to most people, and could, in fact, be
dangerous to some. With so many
choices, it's sometimes difficult to

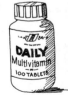

decide whether you need a particular supplement, and if so, which brand to buy. *The Everything® Vitamins Mini Book* was written to provide you with a better understanding of the research behind some of the more popular vitamin supplements, and to help you figure out which, if any, supplements are right for you.

When discussing nutrients and the appropriate levels at which to consume them, a number of standards, requirements, and recommendations are invariably mentioned—and with them, an alphabet soup of abbreviations. Here is a list of the most common abbreviations used in this book:

**Food and Drug Administration (FDA).** The U.S. Food and Drug Administration is a public health agency in charge of protecting the American consumer. It's the FDA's job to see that all food,

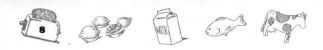

cosmetics, medicines, and medical devices are safe and effective—and won't hurt us. The FDA also monitors all of these products to ensure that they are labeled truthfully, with useful information that will enable people to use them properly.

**Recommended Dietary Allowance (RDA).** The RDAs are the amounts of nutrients that are needed to prevent disease and maintain basic body functions. RDAs are intended to meet the nutrient requirements of nearly all healthy people in certain age and gender groups (as well as during pregnancy and lactation).

The RDAs are set by the Food and Nutrition Board (FNB), a committee of highly regarded nutrition and health professionals who consult to the Institute of Medicine, a section of the National Academy of Sciences (NAS). The

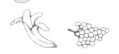

NAS is a private, nonprofit group of scholars that was mandated by Congress in 1863 to advise the federal government on scientific and technical matters.

To set the RDAs, the FNB first determines the least amount of the nutrient needed to prevent deficiency, and then determines the "ceiling" amount or the most that can be consumed— above which health problems occur. Then, a number is selected somewhere between the two limits that provides the body with a reserve amount of the nutrient, but not too much.

The RDAs allow a cushion, calling for more than the average person really needs to stay healthy. That way, if your intake falls short of the RDA amount—for weeks or even a few months— you won't become deficient. RDAs are supposed to be used as goals for dietary intake. People who eat a varied diet generally meet these goals for most nutrients, although there are exceptions, as noted in this book.

**Dietary Reference Intake (DRI).** The FNB has recently completed a new series of dietary recommendations called Dietary Reference Intakes, or DRIs. The DRIs expand on and replace the RDAs. In developing the DRIs, the FNB carefully reviews each nutrient (and other food components that affect human health) not only to establish how much of a nutrient is needed to prevent classical deficiencies (as is done with RDAs), but to determine the nutrient's role in chronic disease, developmental disorders, and other health problems. DRIs are "umbrella" categories, which take into account the RDA values as goals for intake, but also include three new

types of reference values: Estimated Average
Requirement, Adequate Intake, and Tolerable
Upper Intake Level.

**Estimated Average Requirement (EAR).** The EAR
is the amount of a nutrient that is estimated to
meet the nutrient needs of *half* (50 percent) of the
healthy people in certain age and gender groups.
This is done in order to keep the RDA, which
meets the needs of nearly all (97 to 98 percent) of
healthy people, conservatively low. If an EAR
cannot be determined, no RDA is proposed.

**Adequate Intake (AI).** When not
enough is known about a nutrient to
set an EAR or RDA, an AI is established instead. The AI is based on
the observed nutrient intake or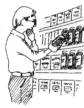

12

experimentally determined estimates of nutrient intake by groups of people. For example, the AI for nutrients for infants aged four to six months is based on the nutrients supplied in breastmilk. Like the RDA, the AI is intended to be a goal of intake for healthy people. When an AI is used, it's an indication that further research is needed in order to more accurately determine the human requirements for that nutrient.

**Tolerable Upper Intake Levels (UL).** The UL is, as one might expect, the highest level of a daily nutrient intake that is likely to pose no risks of adverse health effects to almost all individuals in the general population. The UL is definitely not intended to be a recommended level of intake—there is no established benefit of consuming nutrients at the UL limit.

13

   In some cases UL values could not be established, such as with infants. Of course, this doesn't mean that the body can tolerate chronic, excessive intakes of these nutrients, only that there is a lack of information. When there is a lack of data, it generally pays to be cautious in terms of consumption of these nutrients.

**United States Recommended Daily Allowance (USRDA).** These are just simplified versions of the RDAs that were traditionally used for food labeling purposes. These are being phased out and replaced with Recommended Dietary Intake (RDI) values.

**Daily Value (DV).** The DV recommendations appear on food labels and are a combination of two other standards: the Daily Recommended

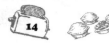

Values, or DRVs (which cover recommendations for fat, carbohydrate, fiber, protein, cholesterol, sodium, and potassium based on a daily intake of 2,000 calories) and the Recommended Dietary Intakes, or RDIs (which replace the old USRDAs). The DV is not the same as the RDA—it isn't as up-to-date. The government has delayed requiring updated label information on supplements until all scientific reviews on RDAs are completed, which is not expected before the year 2005.

**Recommended Dietary Intake (RDI).**
Considered to be the international version of the RDAs, these standards are set by the World Health Organization.

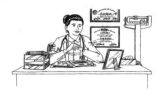

# Supplements: An Overview

With so many different vitamin supplements on the market, and so many advertisements for these products in newspapers and magazines and on television and radio, you might think supplements were essential for good health. The fact of the matter is, although vitamins are necessary for good health, the majority can be obtained from a well-balanced diet.

Can a supplement or two make up for missed nutrients in the diet? Not according to the experts, many of whom believe that

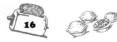

supplements won't fix a bad diet. Unfortunately, many consumers disagree. A number of surveys indicate that roughly 72 percent of those who take vitamin and mineral supplements do so as a type of "insurance." In the American Dietetic Association's national public opinion survey, *Nutrition and You: Trends 2000*, 38 percent of Americans agreed with the statement, "Taking vitamin supplements is necessary to ensure good health." This is up 11 percent from 1993.

So what's a person to do? Are supplements really necessary? Yes and no—it depends on the situation. Given the current information on food intakes in this country, it's safe to say that most people could stand some improvements to their diets—especially in the fruit and vegetable area. And while it's best to get nutrients

from food first, you might want to consider
the following:

- A *multivitamin* providing no more than 100
  to 200 percent of the RDA for most nutrients is probably not a bad idea. In fact,
  some research shows that a basic multi can
  help strengthen the immune system and
  reduce infections in older people.
- Many people, especially women, should
  consider taking a *calcium* supplement
  (most multivitamins do not contain
  enough—if any—calcium because it would
  make the pill too large) if they're not consuming the equivalent of four cups of milk
  per day. And, since vitamin D is necessary
  for calcium absorption, be sure to take a
  multivitamin with D.

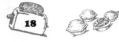   

- *Folic acid* is a must for women of child-bearing age. Get it either through forti-fied foods or a supplement—most multivitamins contain the recommended 400 micrograms.
- Everyone over the age of 50 should con-sider supplementing with *vitamin B$_{12}$*. Some experts recommend 25 micrograms per day; however, most multivitamins only provide 6 micrograms. Be sure to look for one that meets the higher B$_{12}$ level, or think about taking a separate B$_{12}$ supplement.
- An estimated 30 to 40 percent of adults over the age of 50 have borderline *vitamin D* deficiency. Look for a multivitamin that provides 400 International Units (IU). If you're over 70 and get little or no sun,

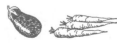

make sure you're getting 600 IU a day of vitamin D.

- Some experts suggest taking 200 to 400 IU a day of *vitamin E.*

# Buying a Supplement

This book provides the reader with general reference information regarding the use and benefits of many different supplements. Once you've become familiar with which supplements might be appropriate for you, you might be tempted to run right out and purchase them. However, it pays to do a little preparation first, so that you'll be sure the supplements you select will be the right ones for you.

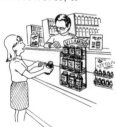

**NOTE:** *The first step to take before actually purchasing supplements is to see your doctor. See "Discuss It with Your Doctor" for specific questions to ask your doctor about your health and the supplements you're interested in taking.*

## Where to Buy Supplements

Supermarkets, drug stores, health food stores, mail-order catalogs, and online outlets are all good sources for dietary supplements, though the selection may be better online or through mail order. Comparison shopping for the most inexpensive supplement (all other things being equal) is wise, as prices can vary widely, and the most expensive supplement isn't necessarily the best. In fact, most manufacturers obtain their vitamins and minerals from the same few sources, so they're all comparable. What may differ is the quality of manufacture, the form, and the extras included in the supplement, such as herbs, enzymes, and phytochemicals—which may or may not be effective or desirable.

In general, store-brand supplements—especially those from larger chains—are often the best bargain and are equal in quality to the higher-priced supplements advertised on television or available from specialty outlets. The least you can expect to pay for a multivitamin and mineral supplement is $1 to $5 for a one-month supply (one tablet per day). When comparing prices online, be sure to factor in shipping and handling charges.

Check that the supplement manufacturer uses Good Manufacturing Practices (GMPs) before purchasing their products. GMPs ensure

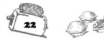

that the product and the potency level match what's indicated on the label. If the label has the seal of the National Nutritional Foods Association, it means that the manufacturer meets the association's standards for quality.

ConsumerLab.com, an independent testing lab, tests products for the presence and the levels of compounds that have been proven effective in clinical research. Those that pass the test are published on their Web site. Also, manufacturers of passing product brands can print the ConsumerLab quality seal on their labels and accompanying product literature.

## Choosing a Supplement Form

This book lists the most common forms available for each supplement. Capsules and tablets are the preferred form for

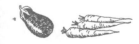

most people since they're easily stored and easily consumed. They're also the most widely available, but there are a variety of other supplement forms that you may want to investigate.

- *Tablets.* Tablets, or their capsule-shaped cousins called "caplets," contain the nutrient itself plus some additives that provide color, help the tablet keep its shape, and break down easily in the body. Talc is a common additive that keeps the ingredients flowing easily during the tableting (or encapsulation) stage of production. In the tiny amounts added to the supplement, talc should not pose any health threat. Tablets are sometimes available in chewable form— for children or those who can't swallow easily. Sublingual tablets are made to be held in the mouth under the tongue until dissolved. Tablets can be stored for long periods of time in a cool, dry location.

- *Capsules.* Capsules tend to have fewer additives because the ingredients don't have to hold their shape as tablets and caplets do. The fat-soluble vitamins A, D, and E are frequently available in "softgel" capsules, which are essentially liquid-containing capsules. Capsules are easily stored for long periods of time in a cool, dry location.

- *Powders.* Powdered supplements are ideal for those who have a hard time swallowing pills, as they can be mixed with beverages or food. However, not many supplements are available in this form. Powders have fewer additives than tablets and capsules. For this reason, people who

are allergic to some additives find powdered supplements more agreeable.
Powders are frequently less expensive than
tablets or capsules. Storage time varies on
powder, but be sure to keep all powders
covered tightly so they're not affected by
humidity in the air.

- *Liquids.* Liquid vitamins can be swallowed
  as is, or mixed with beverages or food.
  Liquids are common for infants' and
  young children's supplements. Liquid supplements may be more quickly absorbed
  by the body, but that doesn't mean the
  nutrients they contain are better absorbed
  or more available to the body. Isotonic
  liquid products supposedly provide
  the nutrients in a similar concentration to that found in the body's

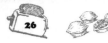
cells, which makes them better absorbed.
However, there is no scientific evidence
that isotonic liquids are absorbed any better
than regular liquids, tablets, or capsules.

- *Lozenges.* Although not a very popular
  form, lozenges are available for some
  supplements, such as zinc. Lozenges
  are supposed to be held in the mouth
  to dissolve slowly.

## How to Read a Supplement Label

Following are some terms you'll need to be
familiar with in order to understand supplement
labels and compare products:

- *Disease claim.* A statement that links the
  supplement to a disease or health condition,

such as calcium and osteoporosis. These
are rarely found on labels, since
the FDA only allows a few supplements
to carry these claims.

- *Directions.* Guidelines for when and how to
  take the supplement, and how much to take.

- *Expiration date.* The date when the supplement may start to lose its potency. It's a
  good idea to finish the product before the
  expiration date, although it isn't dangerous
  to take a product that's passed its expiration
  date (unless the manufacturer indicates otherwise on the label).

- *High potency.* This term may be used to
  describe a single nutrient when it is present
  at 100 percent or more of the Daily Value.
  For multi-ingredient or combination products,
  two-thirds of the nutrients for which the DV

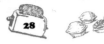

is known must be present at 100 percent or more of the DV, and these nutrients must be specifically named on the label.

- *Ingredients.* Everything that's contained in the supplement will be listed in order of decreasing weight. However, if an ingredient is cited in the "Supplement Facts" panel, it does not have to be included in the ingredients list.

- *Miscellaneous certification insignia.* There are a few patented certification insignia owned by specific manufacturers that may appear on labels. These insignia generally indicate that the products have passed tests for consistency between batches and pills.

- *Serving size.* The manufacturer's suggested serving expressed in terms of the supplement's form, such as "1 tablet." All numerical values listed on the "Supplement Facts" panel are for that specified serving size.

- *Storage advice.* A proper storage place for most supplements is a cool, dry location—not in the bathroom (too hot and damp) or the refrigerator (too cold and damp). Any unusual directions for storage will be stated on the label.

- *Structure/function claim.* This statement indicates the benefit of taking the product and relates it to the body or general health status, such as "aids digestion" or "helps maintain flexible joints." Such claims must also be accompanied on the label by a disclaimer that says that FDA has not evaluated the claim and that the product is not intended to diagnose, treat, cure, or prevent any disease.

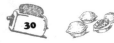   

- *USP.* The abbreviation for the United States Pharmacopeia, an independent body of experts that sets the standards for purity and potency for drugs, supplements, and some herbs. A product that says "USP" on the label indicates that the manufacturer has voluntarily tested the product and found it to comply with USP standards for purity, strength, disintegration, and dissolution.

## Discuss It with Your Doctor

When it comes to dietary supplements, it pays to be cautious. Supplements provide the body with extra nutrients that for some people are beneficial, but for others may be harmful—even deadly. Schedule a physical and use the appointment time to ask your doctor's advice about supplements.

Come prepared—make a list of your questions. Don't be embarrassed to bring a written list or take notes during your discussion. It shows you are serious about getting the information you need to make an informed decision.

In particular, be sure to discuss the following:

- *Any symptoms you may have that suggest a health problem or illness.*
- *Any specific health problems or conditions you have that may cause certain supplements to be dangerous to you.*
- *Medications.* Both prescribed and over-the-counter medications, as well as herbal products, may interact with supplements in ways that can be dangerous. Be sure your doctor knows about all of the medications you are taking.

- *Timing of supplements.* Are there certain times when it isn't advisable to take the supplements you're interested in, because of a medical treatment or health condition? Are there specific times of day when you should take supplements because of potential interactions with medications or other supplements?

- *Dosage.* Dosages can vary according to body weight, sex, severity of the problem you're trying to alleviate or prevent, and other factors. Don't assume that the dosages suggested in this book or on a product label are appropriate for you.

- *Duration of supplement use.* Depending on what supplements you're interested in taking and why, you may be advised to limit the length of time that you take a supplement or combination of supplements.

Although the number of doctors who believe that dietary supplements are "useless and a complete waste of money" seems to be slowly dwindling, there are still many who take this view and advise their patients to avoid supplements completely. Most medical schools teach students very little about nutritional therapy, so your doctor may just be uninformed about supplements and their uses. In either case, don't go it alone. Seek out a doctor who is more receptive or informed about supplements.

Naturopathic doctors (they use the initials "N.D." after their names) are not licensed in most states but do undergo extensive graduate-level training in nutrition, supplements, and herbal medicine. If you want to consult with an N.D., it's best to choose one who has graduated from an accredited school (check with the American Association of Naturopathic Physicians).

Registered Dietitians (they use the initials "R.D." after their names) are another good source of information and guidance regarding dietary supplements. Although nutritionists do not undergo the same level of training that R.D.s do, and there are no licensing requirements for them, some are still good sources of information. You may want to look for those with doctorate degrees; these use the initials "Ph.D." after their names. A pharmacist with a doctorate degree ("Pharm.D.") can also provide information about side effects and interactions, but may not be well versed in the benefits and uses of dietary supplements.

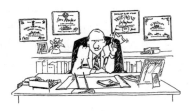

# Guidelines for Using Supplements

You've consulted with your doctor and purchased your supplements; now you need a few pointers about using supplements safely and effectively.

## Don't Exceed the Recommended Dosage

This book gives recommended dosages for some supplements and suggests that you consult your doctor about the appropriate dosages for others. Erring on the side of caution and taking less of a supplement is always wiser than taking more in hopes that it will work better. In general, start with the lowest effective dosage and work up from there if necessary. Megadoses, or extremely high dosages of supplements, should not be taken unless advised and supervised by a physician.

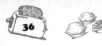

## Check Your Reaction to the Supplement

Some supplements (or ingredients contained in them) may disagree with you or cause an adverse or allergic reaction. Be aware of how you feel, taking note of any symptoms that might be related to the supplement you're taking. If an adverse reaction occurs, stop taking the supplement immediately and contact your doctor.

## Evaluate Your Progress

Not all supplements work for everyone. If you've taken the supplement for the recommended amount of time and you still haven't noticed improvement of your symptoms or health problem, stop taking it and consult your doctor.

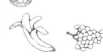

# Children and Vitamins

Like adults, children need a wide variety of
vitamins, minerals, and other nutrients in order
to be healthy. And, as with adults, food is the
primary source of these nutrients. According to
the American Academy of Pediatrics, a healthy
child who eats a balanced diet based on the
Food Guide Pyramid should meet all requirements for essential vitamins and minerals.
Periods of rapid growth, such as infancy and
adolescence, usually require a little more food
but don't necessitate supplements.

Pediatricians may prescribe supplements for
children who have medical conditions that
decrease nutrient absorption, or for children who
follow strict vegetarian diets. Occasionally a liquid
iron supplement will be prescribed for children
who are iron-deficient. *But for most kids—even*

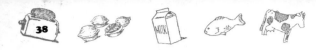

*those who seem to eat unbalanced meals or little food at all—vitamin and mineral supplements are seldom necessary.* Over time, children manage to get the nutrients they need, provided that they're given a variety of foods from which to choose.

Sometimes parents give children a daily multivitamin as a form of nutritional "insurance." Generally, a multivitamin supplement that provides no more than 100 percent of the RDA for nutrients for the child's age is considered safe. It's important to realize, however, that if a child's diet isn't healthy to begin with, supplements won't make it right—they can't make up for too much sugar, too little fiber, or too much fat.

***Never*** give a child any supplement (even a regular multivitamin) designed for adults—they contain too much of certain nutrients that can

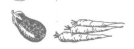

be dangerous for children. Children's vitamin formulas contain the appropriate amounts of nutrients for them, but to be safe, check with the child's pediatrician before giving a child any type of vitamin or mineral supplement. If your child can't chew the vitamin, crush it into smaller pieces to avoid choking. Finally, keep *all* supplements out of reach of children—preferably in a locked cabinet. Young children can mistake them for candy, or may like the taste so much that they overdose on them. If you suspect your child has overdosed on any supplement, call for medical assistance immediately.

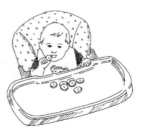

**Part 2**

# Vitamins: Essential Nutrients for Life

## Vitamin A

Vitamin A, the first fat-soluble vitamin to be discovered (in 1913), is the general name given to a family of compounds called retinoids (i.e., retinol, retinal, and retinoic acid). We obtain the vitamin A we need primarily through our diet. However, the body can also convert some carotenoids—yellow, orange, and red pigments in foods—into vitamin A. There are more than 600 different carotenoids in nature, but not all are provitamins—carotenoids that turn into vitamin A in the body. Approximately 90 percent of the vitamin A in the body is stored in the liver.

Vitamin A is believed to be one of the most versatile fat-soluble vitamins because of its role in a number of important body processes. It is important for growth, reproduction, proper bone development, healthy skin, and the immune system. It's also necessary for healthy mucous membranes (the smooth linings of the mouth, stomach, intestines, lungs, etc.). Too little vitamin A, for instance, can lead to a lack of mucus in the eye, causing drying and hardening of the cornea, which can result in blindness.

Vitamin A can be found in a variety of foods, including liver, beef, baked sweet potatoes, raw carrots, cooked spinach, butternut squash, cantaloupe, dried apricots, 2 percent milk, cooked broccoli, egg yolk, cheddar cheese, peaches, baked halibut, butter, and fortified margarine.

## The Benefits of Vitamin A

*Vitamin A and Vision*

Although many of us know that vitamin A is important for vision, most people don't know why. Vitamin A makes up the visual pigments in the eye. One of the earliest signs of vitamin A deficiency is night blindness—or the slow recovery of vision after flashes of bright lights at night. This occurs because there is an insufficient amount of retinal (vitamin A) available to regenerate the pigments bleached by the light.

*Vitamin A and Skin*

Vitamin A also plays a role in healthy skin. Both natural and synthetic forms of the vitamin, such as isotretinoin (trade name Accutane), are regularly used in the treatment of skin disorders including acne and psoriasis. Individuals undergoing retinoid, or vitamin A, therapy are monitored closely to avoid side effects of vitamin A toxicity such as abnormal blood lipid levels, liver toxicity, and birth defects.

*Vitamin A and Other Potential Benefits*

There are a number of alleged benefits of vitamin A supplements, but the scientific research to support such claims is preliminary, contradictory, or significantly lacking at this time. Examples of such uses include the treatment of breast cancer with a retinoid derivative called 4-hydroxyphenylretinamide (4-HPR, Fenretinide) and the use of vitamin A in skin creams to reduce or prevent wrinkling.

## When to Supplement with Vitamin A

Most Americans get enough vitamin A from their diet. The

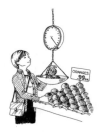

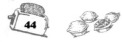   
USDA Continuing Survey of Food Intakes by Individuals in 1994–96 showed an average intake of 1,133 micrograms RE (Retinol Equivalent) of vitamin A for males aged 20 and older, and 982 micrograms RE for females aged 20 and older. The recommended intake for vitamin A for adult males is 900 micrograms per day, and 700 micrograms for adult females.

Vitamin A deficiency is not a common problem in the United States. For that reason, vitamin A is not recommended for children in the United States. However, children, especially those in undeveloped countries, are at an increased risk because they have not yet built up their stores of vitamin A in the liver.

One of the earliest signs of too little vitamin A is night blindness—because of its role in vision. It is estimated that of the 500,000 children worldwide who become blind each year, as many as 70 percent do so because of a vitamin A deficiency. Symptoms of severe vitamin A deficiency can result in abnormal appearance and function of skin, lung, and intestinal tissues.

Although too little vitamin A can pose a problem, too much can be just as devastating. Symptoms of extremely high doses of vitamin A (greater than 200,000 micrograms RE in adults) can include nausea, vomiting, dizziness, blurred vision, muscular uncoordination, and increased cerebrospinal pressure. Chronic high intakes (as much as 10 times the RDA), on the other hand, can result in hair loss, liver damage, bone and muscle pain, headache, and increased blood lipid (fat) levels.

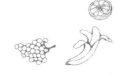

*Vitamin A Toxicity and Osteoporosis*

The highest incidence of osteoporotic fractures (fractures due to bones that are brittle and
porous) in humans is in Northern Europe, where
dietary intake of vitamin A is unusually high. The
average dietary intake of vitamin A in the
Swedish adult population is 1.3 to 1.6 milligrams
per day. And in Norway, intakes can average 1.5
to 2.0 milligrams per day. As a result, researchers
studied a group of 422 women in Sweden,
between the ages of 28 and 74 years. Interestingly,
they found that vitamin A intake was negatively
associated with bone mineral density. In other
words, for every 1-milligram increase in daily
intake of dietary retinol, the risk of hip
fractures increased by 68 percent.
When comparing intakes greater than
1.5 milligrams per day to intakes less
than 0.5 milligrams per day, those with

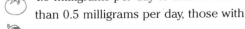

higher intakes had 10 percent less bone mineral density in the neck, 14 percent less at the lumbar spine, and 6 percent less for the whole body. Additionally, the risk of hip fractures was doubled in the higher intake group. The researchers concluded that consuming double the recommended daily amount of vitamin A may dramatically increase the risk of osteoporosis.

*Vitamin A Toxicity and Birth Defects*

Women who are pregnant and take supplements containing more than two-and-a-half times the RDA for vitamin A (more than 10,000 IU a day) have two-and-a-half times the risk of having a baby with defects, compared to women who don't overdose. Moreover, the women who take large amounts of vitamin A are five times more likely to have a baby with a cranial neural crest defect—or a defect resulting in a cleft palate, heart

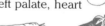

48

abnormalities, and brain damage. Because vitamin
A is involved in the growth and development of a
healthy fetus, too much A, even stored in the
mother's body just before she becomes pregnant,
can wreak havoc. In fact, excess vitamin A poses
the most danger two weeks *before* conception
and during the first two months of pregnancy.
The RDA for pregnant women is 750–770 RE or
approximately 2,500 IU. A single vitamin A supplement, and some multivitamins, can easily contain more than 10,000 IU. Prenatal vitamins
contain as much as 5,000 IU per dose.

## Vitamin B₆ (Pyridoxine)

Vitamin B₆, or pyridoxine (peer-i-DOX-een), was
first discovered in 1938. A water-soluble vitamin,
B₆ is found primarily in muscle and exists in

three interchangeable forms—pyridoxine, pyridoxal, and pyridoxamine. It is one of the most versatile cofactors (essential components of enzymes) of about 120 enzymes (substances that speed up chemical reactions in the body). Vitamin $B_6$ is essential for glucose (blood sugar) production, fat and protein metabolism, and the production of both niacin (another B vitamin) and hemoglobin.

Vitamin $B_6$ can be found in a number of common foods, including liver, beef, chicken, bananas, pistachios, California avocados, mashed potatoes, baked halibut, baked pork chops, sunflower seed kernels, cooked brown rice, dried prunes, 2 percent milk, orange juice, oatmeal, and white bread.

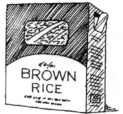

BROWN RICE

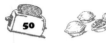

50

# The Benefits of Vitamin B$_6$

*Vitamin B$_6$ and Heart Disease*

Vitamin B$_6$, in conjunction with folate (another B vitamin) and vitamin B$_{12}$, helps to lower blood levels of homocysteine, a risk factor for heart disease. In the Framingham Heart Study, individuals with the lowest vitamin B$_6$ intakes had higher levels of blood homocysteine.

Also, findings from the Nurses' Health Study showed that women with the highest intakes of vitamin B$_6$ and folate had a lower risk of coronary heart disease than women with lower intakes of these vitamins.

*Vitamin B$_6$ and Carpal Tunnel Syndrome*

Over the past 20 years or so, a number of case reports and small studies have suggested that vitamin B$_6$ deficiency might lead to carpal tunnel syndrome (CTS), a painful wrist condition usually linked to repetitive motion injuries. Some researchers believe vitamin $B_6$ may be involved in CTS because of its important role in nerve function.

Although many doctors and CTS sufferers became $B_6$ advocates, no controlled studies have tested the $B_6$ theory. The first study to do so, involving 125 factory workers, found no connection between blood levels of the vitamin and wrist symptoms. Moreover, deficiency of vitamin $B_6$ is rare, and too much of the vitamin can cause severe nerve damage. People with CTS who take the recommended megadoses of $B_6$ (as much as 1,000 milligrams per day) may be putting themselves at risk, since studies have shown that nerve damage can occur with doses as low as 200 milligrams per day.

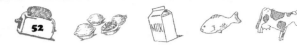

*Vitamin B$_6$ and Premenstrual Syndrome*

For years many women have taken vitamin B$_6$ supplements to relieve premenstrual syndrome (PMS). However, in a recent review of 25 published studies, although B$_6$ fared better than a placebo, researchers found that there was not enough evidence to warrant a recommendation for using megadoses of B$_6$ in the treatment of PMS. Furthermore, because of the potential for toxicity, the researchers concluded that at the moment, there is no rationale for giving vitamin B$_6$ in doses greater than 100 milligrams per day. It may turn out that doses as low as 50 milligrams per day can relieve premenstrual symptoms.

*Vitamin B$_6$ and Other Potential Benefits*

In a study of 70 healthy middle-to-older-age men, those with the highest blood levels of

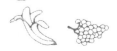

vitamin $B_6$ (similar to that seen with a healthy diet) performed the best on memory tests. Although the results are promising, more research is needed. A number of studies have also looked at the effects of exercise on vitamin $B_6$ status, metabolism, and physical performance, but effects, if any, have been small.

Finally, researchers are also looking at a potential role for vitamin $B_6$ in the treatment of autism. Many children with the disease have been given large doses of vitamin $B_6$ and magnesium. In one study researchers observed positive responses in children receiving as much as 3,000 milligrams of $B_6$ per day. Unfortunately, no other studies have shown similar results. Children being treated with large levels of $B_6$ should

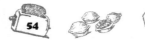

be closely monitored by a physician, because toxicity is a concern.

## When to Supplement with Vitamin B$_6$

National food surveys show that the median daily intake of vitamin B$_6$ in the United States by men is nearly 2 milligrams, and for women it's about 1.5 milligrams—well within the recommended levels. B$_6$ is not recommended for children.

While extreme B$_6$ deficiency is rare (it's never been seen with intakes of 0.5 milligrams or more per day), marginal deficiencies are more likely. Certain groups are at a greater risk of deficiency, including the elderly, alcoholics, and women on high-dose oral contraceptives—although the studies done with contraceptives were conducted when the level of estrogen in

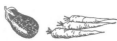

the pill was three to five times higher than the oral agents used today.

When deficiencies occur, they are usually associated with other nutrient deficiencies. For example, since riboflavin is needed for the production of $B_6$, a deficiency in riboflavin could lead to low levels of $B_6$. The earliest symptoms of vitamin $B_6$ deficiency are changes in the nervous system, which can be seen on an EEG (electroencephalogram). Severe deficiency may result in seizures, dermatitis, glossitis (smooth tongue), cheilosis (cracking of corners of the mouth), stomatitis (inflammation of the mouth), irritability, and anemia.

Vitamin $B_6$ supplementation has been used in the treatment of, or in an attempt to prevent, a number of diseases, including Down syndrome, autism, gestational diabetes (diabetes

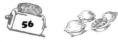

during pregnancy), premenstrual syndrome, CTS, and diabetic neuropathy. However, $B_6$ supplementation has been of limited benefit in these circumstances. And in some cases, such as the treatment of premenstrual syndrome, supplementing with $B_6$ has resulted in a small number of cases of neurotoxicity (which can cause a loss of sensation in hands and feet and an inability to walk) and photosensitivity. These symptoms are usually seen when doses above 500 milligrams per day are used on a chronic basis.

## Vitamin $B_{12}$ (Cobalamin)

Vitamin $B_{12}$, or cobalamin (pronounced co-BALL-uh-min), was first discovered in 1948. Roughly 50 percent of this water-soluble vitamin is stored in the liver and the other half is transported to other tissues. Vitamin $B_{12}$ serves as a cofactor

for two different enzymes. It is necessary for
normal blood formation and neurological
function. Vitamin $B_{12}$ also maintains the sheath,
or covering, that surrounds and protects nerve
fibers and promotes their normal growth.

Vitamin $B_{12}$ can be found in many kinds
of seafood, including clams, oysters,
Dungeness crab, tuna, and halibut,
as well as in beef, liver, milk,
yogurt, pork chops, frankfurters,
eggs, chicken, and ice cream.

## The Benefits of Vitamin $B_{12}$

*Vitamin $B_{12}$ and Heart Disease*

Vitamin $B_{12}$, in conjunction with folate
(another B vitamin) and vitamin $B_6$, helps to
lower blood levels of the amino acid homocysteine, a risk factor for heart disease.

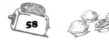

*Vitamin B$_{12}$ and HIV/AIDS*

There is a high prevalence of low vitamin B$_{12}$ levels in people with HIV. In one study, researchers found that individuals with low B$_{12}$ blood levels had a faster progression from HIV to AIDS, compared to those with adequate B$_{12}$ blood levels. In fact, low blood levels of vitamin B$_{12}$ were associated with a nearly twofold increase in risk of progression to AIDS. However, whether or not B$_{12}$ supplementation would slow the progression of the disease is not yet known.

*Vitamin B$_{12}$ and Depression*

In new research from the Women's Health and Aging Study, older women with vitamin B$_{12}$ deficiency appear to be more prone to depression. Experts studied 700 women aged 65 and older, and those with a B$_{12}$ deficiency were more than twice as likely to suffer from severe depression than women without a deficiency. Evidently, a lack of $B_{12}$ may cause a buildup or alteration of chemicals in the brain involved with mood.

*Vitamin $B_{12}$ and Other Potential Benefits*

There are a number of other potential benefits of $B_{12}$ supplements, including the treatment of Alzheimer's disease and dementia, sleep disorders, and diabetic neuropathy. However, further research is needed in these areas.

## When to Supplement with Vitamin $B_{12}$

National food surveys indicate that the median daily intake of vitamin $B_{12}$ in the United States by men is approximately 5 micrograms and the median intake for women is about 3.5 micrograms—well within the recommended levels.

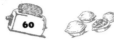

The RDA is 2.4 micrograms for adults. $B_{12}$ is not recommended for children.

There are, however, a number of conditions that may cause deficiencies of vitamin $B_{12}$. Individuals who suffer from malabsorption syndrome of any cause will most likely need extra vitamin $B_{12}$. Diseases/conditions requiring supplementation under a doctor's care include post stomach surgery, pernicious anemia, post-gastric bypass surgery, Crohn's disease, and HIV patients with chronic diarrhea. Treatment usually involves monthly intramuscular injections of 100 micrograms of vitamin $B_{12}$. In addition, the National Academy of Sciences has recommended that individuals over the age of 50 meet their RDA mainly by consuming foods fortified with the synthetic form of $B_{12}$ or a supplement containing vitamin $B_{12}$.

*Vitamin B₁₂ and Pernicious Anemia*

Vitamin $B_{12}$ requires an "intrinsic factor"—a compound made inside the body—for absorption from the intestinal tract into the bloodstream. This intrinsic factor is made in the stomach, where it attaches itself to the vitamin and carries it to the small intestine to be absorbed.

Certain people have a defective gene for intrinsic factor in their genetic makeup, so they can't make it in their bodies. This defect usually becomes evident in midlife. If the intrinsic factor is missing, vitamin $B_{12}$ cannot be absorbed from the diet and deficiency occurs. When this happens, or when the stomach has been injured and cannot produce enough intrinsic factor, $B_{12}$ must be provided via injections in order to bypass the stomach.

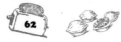

Vitamin $B_{12}$ deficiency, or pernicious anemia, is a type of anemia characterized by large, immature red blood cells identical to those seen in folate deficiency. Symptoms include decreased energy and exercise tolerance, shortness of breath, fatigue, and palpitations. Left untreated, pernicious anemia can lead to a creeping paralysis of the nerves and muscles that begins at the extremities and works up the spine.

Although the symptoms—including the paralysis—can be reversed with vitamin $B_{12}$ treatment, the anemia can be misdiagnosed as a folate deficiency. Folic acid supplements will correct the anemia, but not the damage to the nervous system. For this reason, people over the age of 50 who take folic acid supplements should also take at least 25 micrograms of $B_{12}$ per day, since excess folic acid could mask a potential $B_{12}$ problem.

It is estimated that 10 to 30 percent of people over the age of 50 may develop vitamin $B_{12}$ deficiency due to an inability to absorb the naturally occurring form of $B_{12}$ found in food. Why? Many older people have inadequate gastric (stomach) acid production, which can limit the amount of vitamin $B_{12}$ absorbed. They can, however, absorb synthetic forms of the vitamin, which are found in fortified foods and supplements.

## Vitamin $B_{12}$ and Smoking

Cigarettes have a high cyanide content that can interfere with $B_{12}$ metabolism. In one study, vitamin $B_{12}$ loss in urine was significantly higher among smokers than nonsmokers. However, in other studies the difference has been negligible.

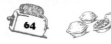

*Vitamin B$_{12}$ and Vegetarians*

Because B$_{12}$ comes from animal products, people who follow a strict vegetarian or vegan diet are at risk for vitamin B$_{12}$ deficiency. This also holds true for babies who are breastfed by vegan mothers. These infants begin to show signs of deficiency at about four months of age. Therefore, infants at risk of B$_{12}$ deficiency should be supplemented with the Adequate Intake (AI) for vitamin B$_{12}$ from birth.

# Vitamin C

Vitamin C, also known as ascorbic acid, is a water-soluble vitamin that aids in wound healing and iron absorption and helps maintain bones, blood vessels, and teeth. Vitamin C helps form

 collagen, a protein that gives structure to bones

and other connective tissues such as gums and blood vessel walls. It also plays an important role in the production of hormones and the amino acid carnitine.

Vitamin C has long been heralded for its antioxidant properties. Antioxidants are special compounds that protect against oxidation, or cellular damage caused by free radicals. Common examples of oxidation in everyday life include the rusting of metal and the browning of fruit. In the human body, oxygen-derived free radicals are highly reactive molecules that are normally produced as a byproduct of metabolism in cells. However, free radicals can also be generated in the body as a result of exposure to sunlight, x-rays, tobacco smoke, car exhaust, and other environmental pollutants. Excessive free-radical formation can overwhelm the body's

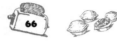

antioxidant defense mechanisms and may lead
to a number of chronic diseases such as
cancer, stroke, diabetes, heart and lung disease,
and cataracts.

Vitamin C can be found in fruits such as
cantaloupe, kiwis, oranges (and orange juice),
mangos, grapefruit, papayas, strawberries, lemons,
and watermelon. It is also found in vegetables
such as peppers, tomatoes, broccoli, cauliflower,
collards, potatoes, and spinach.

## The Benefits of Vitamin C

*Vitamin C and Heart Disease*

As an antioxidant, vitamin C may improve
immune function and reduce the risk of heart
disease by preventing the oxidation of LDL (low-
density lipoprotein or "bad" cholesterol). A
lipoprotein is a molecule that carries fat through

the blood. Research indicates that LDL oxidation increases the risk for plaque formation, which can clog arteries and lead to a heart attack or stroke. Vitamin C also protects vitamin E from oxidation. Research has shown that vitamin E protects against heart disease, too.

Vitamin C may also affect heart health by preventing blood vessels from constricting and thus cutting off blood supply to the heart. This benefit may even be seen in people who already have cardiovascular disease. In one study of individuals with diseased arteries, taking 500 milligrams of supplemental vitamin C per day for a month completely normalized the blood flow in their arteries. A number of studies have also shown that supplementing with 1,000 to 2,000 milligrams of vitamin C per day can help block the

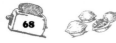   
dangerous artery-destroying effects of the amino acid homocysteine.

### Vitamin C and Blood Pressure

Supplementing with 500 milligrams of vitamin C per day may lower blood pressure according to a recent study. Evidently, vitamin C increases the activity and levels of nitric oxide, which relaxes arteries and lowers blood pressure. Nitric oxide also helps prevent clot formation and plaque buildup on artery walls.

### Vitamin C and Cancer

There is growing evidence that vitamin C may have a protective effect in cancers of the esophagus, mouth, pharynx, stomach, pancreas, cervix, rectum, breast, and lung. The most promising evidence, however, is with stomach cancer. High doses of vitamin C in animals inhibit *H. pylori*, the bacterium that is responsible for most ulcers and possibly an increased risk of stomach cancer. Vitamin C may also protect against cancer by neutralizing free radicals or blocking the formation of nitrosamines. These carcinogenic compounds form when nitrates (found naturally in foods and as food additives) or nitrites (found naturally in saliva) combine with substances called amines in the digestive juices of the stomach.

Interestingly, a recent study suggested that individuals with cancer who take megadoses of vitamin C may actually be hurting themselves rather than helping. It seems that cancer cells contain vitamin C, which may protect them from oxidation. Many cancer treatments, especially radiation, work by causing oxygen damage to cancer cells. Thus, vitamin C may be working against some forms of cancer treatment. Although these

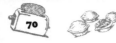   

findings are preliminary, the researchers advise that cancer patients avoid supplementing with more than the RDA for vitamin C.

*Vitamin C and Cataracts*

In its role as an antioxidant, vitamin C is believed to help protect against cataracts. Researchers at Tufts and Harvard universities studied nearly 250 women with no history of cataracts. Those who had been supplementing with vitamin C for at least 10 years had 77 percent fewer early-stage opacities (the first sign of cataracts) and 83 percent fewer moderate opacities than women who did not supplement. Although there is much debate among the experts regarding how much vitamin C is necessary for this protective effect, 150 to 200

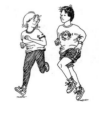

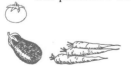

milligrams is the amount needed to saturate eye tissues.

*Vitamin C and Iron Deficiency*

Vitamin C can increase iron absorption, which can be helpful for those with an iron deficiency, or for women, who generally have higher iron needs and low intakes. However, it can be a problem for men, who tend to take in too much iron. In fact, some researchers suspect that iron overload among men may contribute to heart disease and several types of cancer. Too much iron in the body may lead to oxidative reactions that can damage tissues and DNA. More research is needed in this area.

*Vitamin C and Gallbladder Disease*

A recent study indicates that women who don't get enough vitamin C may be at a greater

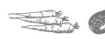

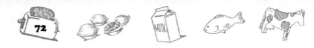

risk for gallbladder disease. Gallstones are often formed when bile, a liquid formed by the liver to help break down fats during digestion, becomes saturated with cholesterol. Vitamin C helps break down cholesterol, preventing it from hardening into gallstones. These stones can grow as large as one inch across and cause severe abdominal pain. In some cases treatment involves removing the gallbladder altogether.

Gallstones affect many more women than men. This may be due, in part, to the fact that estrogen increases the concentration of cholesterol in bile—and most gallstones are made up of cholesterol. The findings from this latest study indicate that women who have higher blood levels of vitamin C and those who take vitamin C supplements have a lower risk of gallstones and gallbladder disease.

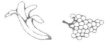

*Vitamin C and Asthma*

Vitamin C may help people with exercise-induced asthma (EIA) breathe more easily. In a well-controlled study from Israel, individuals with EIA were given a single dose of 2,000 milligrams of vitamin C one hour before exercising on a treadmill. The researchers found that ascorbic acid prevented or decreased the severity of wheezing attacks and lung discomfort in over half of the study participants. It appears that vitamin C may protect against damaging oxidants in the lungs.

*Vitamin C and Other Potential Benefits*

There are a number of alleged benefits of vitamin C supplements that have not been proven by scientific research or are still under investigation. One of the more infamous claims for vitamin C is that it prevents colds. Unfortunately, there has not been a study to date that has shown that supplementing with vitamin C can reduce the risk of catching a cold, although it may shorten the duration and/or severity of the cold.

Lead poisoning is a major public health problem in this country. In a recent study, researchers found that high blood levels of ascorbic acid were associated with a decreased prevalence of elevated blood lead levels in adults. If vitamin C does truly affect blood lead levels, vitamin C intake could have public health implications for control of lead toxicity.

Preliminary research has also suggested that supplementing with vitamin C may protect against mental declines following a stroke or other circulatory problems, although much more research is needed. Finally, researchers are also looking at a potential role for vitamin C in the prevention of osteoporosis and periodontal disease.

## When to Supplement with Vitamin C

As long ago as the 1700s, sailors realized that consuming foods with vitamin C could prevent scurvy, or vitamin C deficiency. Although scurvy is rarely seen in developed countries, certain people are at greater risk, including those who consume few fruits and vegetables or abuse alcohol or drugs. In the United States, low vitamin C levels in the blood are more common in men—especially the elderly—than in women and are more prevalent in lower socioeconomic groups.

Symptoms of scurvy include swollen, bleeding gums; loosening of the teeth; hemorrhaging, including bleeding into the joints;

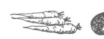

tender and painful extremities; poor wound healing; weakness and fatigue; and psychological disturbances.

For many years experts thought the only use for vitamin C was to prevent scurvy. However, although as little as 10 milligrams of vitamin C per day will prevent deficiency, much higher levels are needed for stress situations such as trauma, wound healing, and infection. Over the years more and more research has shown that vitamin C may be necessary for the prevention of *disease*—not just deficiency.

As a result, the RDA for vitamin C was recently increased to 90 milligrams for adult men and 75 milligrams for adult women. The higher levels were set to achieve maximum saturation of vitamin C in the body without excess loss in the urine. It was also recommended that smokers take in an additional 35 milligrams per day to offset some of the oxidative damage from cigarettes. However, some experts argue that these new levels are not high enough. In a report published in 1999, researchers at the National Institutes of Health suggested raising the recommended intake of vitamin C to 100 to 200 milligrams per day.

The USDA Continuing Survey of Food Intakes by Individuals in 1994–96 showed an average daily intake of 109 milligrams of vitamin C for males aged 20 and older, and 91 milligrams for females aged 20 and older.

Although vitamin C toxicity is not a problem for most people, there are certain groups that are at risk of getting too much of this nutrient. Individuals with kidney disease, for instance, should avoid getting more than the RDA.

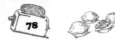   

Additionally, intakes above 250 milligrams per day can cause false-negative results in tests for stool and gastric blood. Therefore, high-dose supplementation with vitamin C should be stopped at least two weeks before physical exams because they may interfere with blood and urine tests.

## Vitamin D

Vitamin D has long been known as "the sun-shine vitamin" because the body can make it when the skin is exposed to sunlight. Actually, what we know as vitamin D really isn't a vitamin at all—it's a steroid hormone. Long ago it was misclassified as a fat-soluble vitamin and the name just stuck. It does have some of the same characteristics of a vitamin; namely, that people

 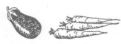

who are not exposed to sunlight need to get vitamin D from food or supplements just as they do for other vitamins. To make matters even more confusing, vitamin D is actually a general term for the many forms of the vitamin. The two major forms are vitamin $D_2$ and vitamin $D_3$, which were discovered in the 1930s.

Vitamin $D_2$ (also called ergocalciferol) is the plant form of the vitamin—the form found in some foods and used most often in supplements. Vitamin $D_3$ (also called cholecalciferol) is the form that's produced when the skin is exposed to sunshine. Some vitamin $D_3$ is stored in the liver and kidneys, some goes to the bones, and the rest goes to the intestines to aid in calcium absorption from food.

Vitamin D can be found in foods such as salmon, milk, sardines, egg yolks, cheddar cheese, and butter.

## The Benefits of Vitamin D

Vitamin D's most important function is to regulate the body's absorption and use of calcium and phosphorus, thereby making this vitamin essential for bone and tooth formation and strength. Since calcium is also necessary for muscle contraction (including the heart muscle) and sending messages along the nerves, vitamin D is important in these areas, too.

### Vitamin D and Osteoporosis

Osteoporosis is a progressive condition characterized by decreased bone density. That is, the mineral content of the bones is diminished, making them brittle, weak, and more likely to break. The condition is most common in women who have gone through menopause, but older men get osteoporosis, too, though it's generally less severe. Although most people think of calcium as being the anti-osteoporosis nutrient, vitamin D's role is also essential.

Bone fractures (often of the hip or spine) in older people are increasingly recognized to be a result of osteoporosis. And for more than 20 years, experts have known that vitamin D deficiency is associated with an increased risk of hip fracture. A recent study conducted at Brigham and Women's Hospital in Boston found that half of the women with hip fractures were deficient in vitamin D.

In some regions of the United States, where sunshine is less abundant and weaker during the winter, researchers have documented measurable loss of bone mineral density in the hips and spines of older people. This is especially troublesome for those who may not be getting adequate amounts of vitamin D from milk products. Researchers from Tufts University found that daily supplements of 500 milligrams of calcium plus 700 IU of vitamin D, taken for three years, decreased the risk of bone fractures in older men and women by 50 percent. A previous study with the same supplements taken over a two-year period resulted in a 43 percent reduction of hip fractures in older women. Experts believe that the main way vitamin D contributes to bone density is by increasing calcium absorption in the small intestine. This ensures an adequate level of calcium in the blood, which can then be deposited in the bone.

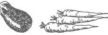

*Vitamin D and Other Potential Benefits*

There is some preliminary evidence that vitamin D supplements may slow the progression of osteoarthritis in the knees. A study of 556 participants showed that, among those people who already had arthritic knees, those who also had low blood levels of vitamin D were three times more likely to experience a worsening of their arthritis than those with higher levels of the vitamin.

There are some reports that link vitamin D deficiency to colon and breast cancers. These two types of cancers are more common among people who live in northern climates, where there's less opportunity to get the vitamin from sunshine. Although these studies are still speculative, what is known is that vitamin D inhibits the growth of cancer cells in test tubes. Currently, a

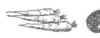

government-funded study called the Women's Health Initiative is looking into the potential role of vitamin D in cancer.

Psoriasis, a chronic disease that results in itchy, red, flaky patches on the skin, can be treated with sunshine and a prescription cream called Dovonex, which contains a form of vitamin D. However, taking vitamin D supplements alone, or using nonprescription creams with vitamin D, won't work.

## When to Supplement with Vitamin D

Surveys indicate that the usual dietary intake of vitamin D in the United States is low—50 to 70 IU per day. Presumably, vitamin D stores are enriched in most people by regular exposure to sunlight, at least during certain times of the year. Recommended intake for vitamin D for males and females aged 51 to 70 is 400 IU, or 600 IU per day if over age 70. Vitamin D is not recommended for infants and children unless supervised by a doctor.

*Vitamin D Deficiency*

The symptoms of vitamin D deficiency include muscle twitching, cramps, and convulsions, as well as aching bones. Conditions that would cause a vitamin D deficiency include severe liver failure, Crohn's disease, and celiac sprue (a malabsorption disorder caused by an intolerance to a protein found in wheat, rye, oats, and barley).

Children who are vitamin D deficient get rickets, which is characterized by short stature, bowlegs or "knock-knees," and deformities of the skull. In the United States, rickets was virtually eliminated by the 1930s because of the fortification of milk with vitamin D. In Europe, however, foods are not fortified with vitamin D, which is why rickets continues to be a health problem in some European countries. Adults who are vitamin D deficient develop osteomalacia, sometimes called "adult rickets." Osteomalacia doesn't cause bone deformities, but it does result in a decrease of the mineral content of the bones, leaving them more prone to fractures. Some people with osteomalacia complain of deep bone pain. Adults over age 50 should consider getting a blood test for vitamin D levels (the form called 25-hydroxyvitamin D) because until a deficiency is quite severe, it's hard to detect. Women should also consider getting a bone mineral density test.

*Older People Need More Vitamin D*

The recommended amounts of vitamin D are difficult to get if one doesn't drink milk or get

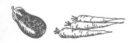

regular exposure to the sun. Older people who are housebound or living in nursing homes and rarely spend any time outside in the sun are particularly at risk for vitamin D deficiency. In fact, experts estimate that up to 40 percent of Americans over the age of 50 are vitamin D deficient. Compared to adults aged 20 to 30, those over age 65 produce four times less vitamin D in their skin. It's recommended that people over age 50 take a multivitamin that contains 400 IU of vitamin D per day, as well as a calcium supplement with added vitamin D (200 IU).

*People in Northern Climates Need More Vitamin D*

The body can store vitamin D (in the fatty tissues and liver) for a long time, so for most people who are outside a lot during sunny months, body stores of the vitamin are probably sufficient to last the winter. However, people who live in the northern United States or other northern regions and consume little vitamin D may be at increased risk for developing vitamin D deficiency. In northern climates, a multivitamin containing 200 IU of vitamin D is recommended to supplement dietary intake in the winter months. Those who reside year-round in cloudy climates such as Seattle or London may also be deficient and should take the same supplement all year long. And, if the diet contains no fortified milk, a higher-dose vitamin D supplement may be necessary to bring intake up to the recommended levels.

*Vitamin D Toxicity*

Reports of vitamin D toxicity from food sources are extremely rare since very few

foods contain much of the vitamin. However, high intakes of fatty fish or milk may put one at risk for vitamin D toxicity. With supplements, the chance of getting too much vitamin D is much greater, especially in people who take more than one vitamin D–containing supplement per day (such as a multivitamin and a calcium-plus-vitamin-D supplement).

The upper limit for vitamin D is 1,000 IU per day for infants and 2,000 IU per day for everyone else, including pregnant or lactating women. At an intake of 3,800 IU per day, hypercalcemia (too much calcium) can occur, since vitamin D facilitates calcium absorption. This condition can cause calcification of the soft tissues including the kidneys, blood vessels, heart, and lungs. In

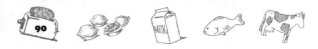

infants, intakes greater than 45 micrograms per day may reduce growth.

Other symptoms of vitamin D toxicity include loss of appetite, nausea, vomiting, thirst, joint pains, muscular weakness, and disorientation. Ironically, getting too much vitamin D can cause bone demineralization and bone loss. Severe vitamin D toxicity can be fatal.

## Vitamin E

Vitamin E, discovered in 1922, is the general name for eight different forms of the vitamin: four tocopherols and four tocotrienols. The tocopherols are the most important, and these are designated alpha, beta, delta, and gamma (i.e., beta-tocopherol). Alpha-tocopherol has the highest biological activity. The tocotrienols are active in the body, but are usually considered less nutritionally important. Tocopherols and tocotrienols are the general names for the two primary chemical structures of vitamin E. Within each group are four forms of the vitamin that differ from each other slightly in chemical structure.

Vitamin E is generally considered the major fat-soluble antioxidant in the blood and body tissues. As such, it is the first line of defense against free radicals—unstable oxygen molecules that can damage body cells and may lead to heart disease, cancer, stroke, and other health problems. (For more information about free radicals, see the vitamin C section.) Vitamin E, which is stored mainly in fat tissue and the liver, is particularly important in the brain and nervous system. Foods that contain vitamin E include toasted wheat germ, almonds, hazelnuts,

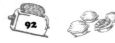

sunflower oil, safflower oil, canola oil, cotton-
seed oil, wheat germ oil, boiled turnip greens,
canned spinach, Italian salad dressing,
anchovies in oil, navy beans, and fried eggs.

## The Benefits of Vitamin E

*Vitamin E and Heart Disease*

Vitamin E could well be considered the
nutrient of the 1990s. That was the decade when
the popularity of the vitamin soared as a result of
evidence from almost 20 population studies that
suggested that people who had a high intake of
vitamin E had a reduced risk of heart disease.
But, population studies can only draw associations—they don't prove true cause and effect.
Intervention trials (also called clinical trials, where
particular treatments are specifically investigated
with carefully selected participants in a controlled

setting) are needed for that—and there haven't been many.

A study in China showed heart benefits from vitamin E supplementation, but the supplements contained more than just vitamin E, so it's unclear which of the ingredients was the most helpful. The Cambridge Heart Antioxidant Study, an intervention trial with 2,002 people, demonstrated that supplementing with vitamin E reduced nonfatal heart attack risk by 77 percent compared to a placebo.

Recently, however, the Heart Outcomes Prevention Evaluation in Canada failed to show that vitamin E supplements decrease the risk of heart disease or stroke. In this study, 9,500 people aged 55 and up who were diagnosed with cardiovascular disease or diabetes (a major risk factor for cardiovascular disease) received either

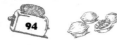

94

a placebo or a 400 IU supplement of vitamin E
daily. After four and a half years, those who took
vitamin E were no less likely than the placebo-
takers to have had a heart attack or stroke, or to
have died from cardiovascular disease. There was
also no difference between the groups in fre-
quency of other heart problems such as angina.
Another study in Italy concluded that 300 IU of
supplemental synthetic (manmade) vitamin E,
taken daily for three and a half years, did not significantly reduce risk of heart attack or stroke in
more than 11,000 men and women.

Why the discrepancy? It may be that vitamin
E only offers protection from cardiovascular
disease in otherwise healthy people—not a
reversal of the condition or a cure. Perhaps, as
the researchers acknowledge, vitamin E may

work best when taken in conjunction with other

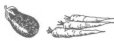

antioxidants. Also, the form of vitamin E may be causing the conflicting results. Some animal studies have shown that gamma-tocopherol (the type found primarily in foods) may be more effective in preventing free radical damage than alpha-tocopherol, the form used most frequently in supplements. In any case, a number of other trials with vitamin E are currently under way, and the overall body of research does indicate some probable benefit from vitamin E supplements.

*Vitamin E and Alzheimer's Disease*

There is a good amount of evidence to suggest that free radical damage to the neurons (nerve cells) is at least partially responsible for the development of Alzheimer's disease. Studies have also shown an association between

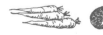

vitamin E and the risk of, or progression of, Alzheimer's disease.

Vitamin E has been shown to prevent free radical damage and delay memory deficits in animal studies. And, a recent human study in which participants took 2,000 IU of vitamin E per day showed that the supplement may slow the functional deterioration that frequently leads to placement in a health-care or long-term care facility. In a two-year study of people with Alzheimer's disease, progression of the disease was slowed when either 2,000 IU of vitamin E (alpha-tocopherol), a drug (10 milligrams Selegiline), or a combination of the two was taken daily. The researchers noted that, compared to those taking a placebo, those in the treatment groups took seven months longer to reach severe dementia, institutionalization, loss of the ability to perform basic activities of living, and death. The combined treatment (drug plus vitamin E) appeared to be just as effective as either component alone.

Although the evidence for vitamin E is promising, it's important to note that such large doses of vitamin E, when taken by healthy people, have not been shown to *prevent* Alzheimer's disease. What's more, the safety and efficacy of supplemental vitamin E taken over many years has not been adequately studied. Whether the risks associated with large doses of vitamin E are worth any possible benefit is a decision that should be made with the help of a personal physician.

*Vitamin E and Cancer*

A number of epidemiological studies suggest that low blood levels or intakes of vitamin E are associated with increased risk of certain types of cancer. Occurrence of cancer of the stomach, esophagus, and cervix seems to be reduced when antioxidant supplements (including vitamin E) are taken for a period of years. Vitamin E supplements have also been associated with lower risk of oral, colon, breast, thyroid, prostate, gastrointestinal tract, lung, and bladder cancers. In many cases, at least 100 IU of vitamin E per day is needed. And, studies seem to indicate that vitamin E is not effective if a person already has cancer. In other words, it doesn't cure or reverse cancer progression, but it may delay or prevent it. However, since most results only show associations between vitamin E and cancer outcomes—not true cause-and-effect relationships—some researchers think it's premature to recommend supplements for the prevention of cancer. What's more, many of these studies used supplements containing a mixture of antioxidants, so it's impossible to say that vitamin E supplements alone will produce similar effects.

*Vitamin E and Cataracts*

A cataract starts off as a cloudy spot on the lens of the eye, which may or may not interfere with vision. As it gets worse, or as more of them develop on the lens, blurred vision, sensitivity to light, and changes in color perception may occur. Although cataract surgery is performed on an outpatient basis and is very successful, preventing cataracts in the first place is even better. Age is still considered the major risk factor in cataract development, which is caused by exposure to ultraviolet radiation (sunlight) that causes oxidation, or free radical damage.

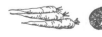

A number of epidemiological studies have suggested an association between cataract development and low blood levels of vitamin E and other antioxidants. For example, in a U.S. study of 112 people, high blood levels of at least two of the three antioxidant nutrients (vitamins E, C, and carotenoids) were associated with a significantly reduced risk of cataract development compared to people with low levels of at least one of the nutrients. Two studies conducted in Finland have shown an association between low vitamin E levels and cataract risk, or the development of cortical lens opacities (cloudy spots on the lens that lead to cataract formation).

Experts suggest that vitamin E will not prevent cataracts, but supplements may delay the onset  and slow the progression of cataract development.

A few animal studies have shown this to be true, but clinical trials with humans are necessary in order to firmly establish vitamin E's efficacy in cataract prevention.

*Vitamin E and Immunity*

Aging is associated with a decline in immune status, which leads to more infections, cancers, and other chronic diseases. A study conducted at the Human Nutrition Research Center on Aging at Tufts University examined the effects of various vitamin E supplements on 78 healthy people aged 65 and older. After four months, those who took 200 milligrams of vitamin E per day had stronger responses to vaccines for hepatitis B and tetanus than those who took the placebo. That is, they created more antibodies to fight off future attacks of the illnesses. Responses for other doses

(60 or 800 milligrams) were not as good. The vitamin E takers also experienced 30 percent fewer infections, and other indicators of immunity were also improved by the supplements. Finally, immune effects were confirmed in people under age 30 as well, with six months of supplementation with 400 IU of vitamin E.

## Vitamin E and Other Potential Benefits

There are many additional areas of vitamin E research, including male infertility, diabetes, skin disorders, circulatory problems, and physical performance (both in athletes and in people who live at high altitudes). Vitamin E supplementation appears somewhat promising for each of these areas, but at the current time the research is preliminary. The use of topical (applied to the skin) vitamin E in treating skin wounds has been investigated for years, with conflicting results. A recent study of 15 people who had skin cancers removed and were treated with either topical vitamin E or a placebo showed that there was no benefit to using the vitamin (the wounds didn't heal faster or scar less). What's more, a third of the participants developed inflamed skin from the vitamin E treatment.

## When to Supplement with Vitamin E

For adults, the recommended amount of daily vitamin E intake is 15 milligrams (22 IU of natural-source vitamin E or 33 IU of the synthetic form) of alpha-tocopherol. According to the USDA Continuing Survey of Food Intakes by Individuals 1994–96, the average reported dietary intake of vitamin E for people aged 31 to 50 years is

7.5 milligrams alpha-tocopherol per day for men and 5.4 milligrams for women—significantly below the recommended amounts. However, this survey probably underestimated actual vitamin E intake because of measurement errors that are common with vitamin E. According to the National Academy of Sciences, real vitamin E intake in the United States and Canada is likely to meet or even exceed the RDA level.

Vitamin E supplements are not recommended for children.

*Vitamin E Deficiency*

A deficiency of vitamin E causes reproductive problems; neurological abnormalities, including diminished reflexes, limb weakness, sensory loss in the arms and legs, and difficulty walking;

immunological abnormalities; and hemolytic anemia (breakdown of red blood cells).

Deficiency is not common, but is known to occur in premature infants with very low birth weights and in people suffering from malnutrition. The most common cause of vitamin E deficiency is fat malabsorption. People who can't absorb fat properly cannot absorb vitamin E well either, since it's a fat-soluble vitamin. Therefore, cystic fibrosis, chronic liver disease, chronic diarrhea, celiac sprue (a condition where food absorption is impaired due to an intolerance to gluten, a protein found in certain grains), short bowel syndrome, and Crohn's disease hamper vitamin E absorption. For people with these conditions, a water-soluble vitamin E supplement is suggested. People who follow a very low-fat, low-calorie diet and those who take cholesterol-lowering drugs may also be at risk for deficiency.

Because vitamin E is stored in the body for long periods of time, it takes several years in adults before blood levels of the vitamin decrease to a deficient range. Neurologic abnormalities may take five to 10 years to appear. However, in children with vitamin E malabsorption from infancy (such as those born with liver diseases), vitamin E deficiency can develop rather early in life, rapidly producing neurologic symptoms if the deficiency is untreated. If corrected in the first few years of life, all symptoms can be reversed or prevented. Once neurologic damage has occurred, vitamin E can produce only limited improvement.

*Vitamin E Toxicity*

Compared with the other fat-soluble vitamins, oral vitamin E supplements produce few side effects and are relatively nontoxic. In adults, large doses may interfere with the absorption of vitamins A and K and cause fatigue, gastrointestinal upset, breast soreness, and thyroid problems. The biggest concern with large amounts of vitamin E relates to the vitamin's blood-thinning effect. Intakes of more than 1,200 milligrams per day, combined with anticoagulant medications, can cause dangerous bleeding. Even on its own, vitamin E can lead to post-surgery bleeding when taken in doses greater than 800 to 1,200 milligrams per day. In premature infants, large doses of vitamin E have caused a number of problems, including an increased risk of infection and gastrointestinal problems.

# Folic Acid

Folic acid, or folate, is a B vitamin that appears
to be protective against certain birth defects,
cancer, and heart disease. Folate is the form
found naturally in foods, and folic acid is the
synthetic form found in fortified foods and supplements. Folate is needed to make DNA, the
carrier of genetic information in all cells.
Rapidly dividing cells, especially in the blood,
the developing fetus, and the lining of the
colon, need folic acid the most. Folate is also
necessary for the production of red blood cells
and protein metabolism, and to convert the
amino acid homocysteine into another amino
acid, methionine. It can be found in foods such
as beef liver, cooked lentils, fortified cereal,
cooked enriched white rice, cooked enriched
macaroni, cooked enriched noodles, cooked

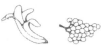

black beans, spinach, cooked asparagus, cooked mustard greens, orange juice, enriched bagels, avocados, raw broccoli, baked potatoes with the skin, and eggs.

## The Benefits of Folic Acid

*Folic Acid and Birth Defects*

In recent years researchers have discovered that folic acid reduces the risk of neural tube defects (NTDs), one of the most serious and common birth defects in the United States. These defects occur in the neural tube, which develops into the spinal cord. If the defect occurs at the top of the tube, the result is fatal, since the baby is born with anencephaly (no brain). If the defect occurs farther down on the tube, the baby is born with spina bifida (an open spine). Damage to the exposed spinal cord usually results in a child who is either wheel-chair bound or on crutches.

Each year, an estimated 2,500 babies are born with these defects, and many additional affected pregnancies result in miscarriage or stillbirth. Since these birth defects occur within the first month of pregnancy—before many women even know they're pregnant—it is important for a woman to have enough folic acid in her system prior to conception. Folic acid, when consumed in adequate amounts by women at least one month prior to and for 6 weeks after conception, can prevent up to 70 percent of these birth defects. The benefits are so great that in 1992 the U.S. Public Health Service recommended that all women of childbearing age consume 400 micrograms of folic acid every day.

*Folic Acid and Down's Syndrome*

In a recent study, researchers found that supplementing with folic acid may also help prevent Down's syndrome, one of the most common developmental disorders in the United States. This syndrome affects nearly 1 in 150 conceptions every year. Although the age of the mother has long been recognized as a risk factor for Down's syndrome, most children with the disorder are born to women under the age of 30.

Down's syndrome is caused by a genetic mutation resulting in an extra chromosome. Previous research suggests that insufficient folate leads to some genetic mutations. The theory is that low folate levels may increase the risk of a genetic mutation leading to Down's syndrome. Although more research is needed, consuming enough folic acid to meet the RDA is the prudent thing to do for all women of childbearing age.

*Folic Acid and Heart Disease*

Folate may also play an important role in reducing the risk for cardiovascular disease. It is involved in controlling blood levels of homocysteine by converting this amino acid into methionine. High levels of homocysteine may increase the risk of heart disease and stroke. In the Physicians' Health Study, men who started out with elevated homocysteine levels were three times as likely to have a heart attack over the next five years.

Previous research indicates that folic acid intakes of 400 micrograms (the current RDA) or more per day may keep homocysteine at stable low levels. The same research suggests that possibly 88 to 90 percent of the population is not consuming enough folate to keep homocysteine levels low. Findings from the Nurses' Health Study showed that women with the highest intakes of folate and vitamin B$_6$ had a lower risk of coronary heart disease than women with lower intakes of these vitamins.

*Folic Acid and Colon Cancer*

A growing body of clinical studies suggests a possible association between low folate status and an increased risk for cancer, with the strongest evidence for colorectal cancer—one of the leading causes of death by cancer in the United States. In findings from the U.S. Nurses' Health Study, women who had been taking a multivitamin with folic acid for at least 15 years had 75 percent less risk of developing colon cancer than those who didn't take multivitamins. Folate from foods also appeared to be protective, but not significantly.

**114**

Similar findings were also seen in men in the U.S. Health Professionals Follow-up Study. Men who reported eating the most folate-rich foods were less likely to develop colon cancer over the next few years. Researchers suspect that folate protects against DNA damage—which can cause cancer.

Researchers are also investigating the protective effects of folate against lung, esophagus, uterine, cervix, and liver cancers. Here, however, more research is needed.

*Folic Acid and Alcohol*

In a recent study of 90,000 women, those who consumed less than 300 micrograms of folate per day and regularly drank alcohol (at least one drink per day) increased their risk of breast cancer by 30 percent, compared to those who drank less than one drink per day.

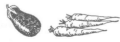

However, breast cancer risk increased by only 5 percent in those who regularly drank alcohol while consuming more than 300 micrograms of folate per day. Apparently, alcohol interferes with folate metabolism, preventing the vitamin from reaching tissue cells, thereby leaving them vulnerable to cancerous changes. Consuming adequate folate helps counteract this effect.

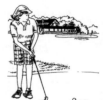

*Folic Acid and Other Potential Benefits*

There are a number of alleged benefits of folic acid supplements, but the evidence to support such claims is very preliminary. One example is the possible use of folic acid to treat depression. Several studies have shown individuals suffering from depression may have low folate levels.

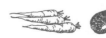

**116**

# When to Supplement with Folic Acid

Folate in food is nearly 50 percent less bioavailable than folic acid in fortified foods and supplements. In fact, folate is one of the few nutrients that is more beneficial in the manmade form than the natural form.

Folate deficiency is one of the most common nutrient deficiencies in the United States and can result in megaloblastic anemia, which is characterized by a reduced number of red blood cells. Side effects of the anemia include weakness, fatigue, headache, irritability, difficulty concentrating, and shortness of breath.

It is not recommended that children take folic acid supplements.

*Folate and Vitamin B$_{12}$ Deficiency*

Folate and vitamin B$_{12}$ work closely together, and a deficiency of either nutrient leads to anemia. However, in the case of vitamin $B_{12}$, deficiency can bring about not only anemia, but nerve damage as well. If a $B_{12}$ deficiency is misdiagnosed as a folate deficiency, folic acid supplements will correct the anemia but not the damage to the nervous system. For this reason, people over the age of 50 who take folic acid supplements should also take at least 25 micrograms of $B_{12}$ per day, since excess folic acid could mask a potential $B_{12}$ deficiency.

## Folate and Alcohol

Surveys of chronic alcoholics suggest that inadequate intake is a major cause of folate deficiency in this group. Additionally, ethanol intake may impair folate absorption and increase folate loss in the urine.

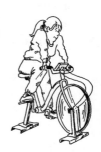

*Folate–Drug Medications*

Methotrexate is an "anti-folate" medication that has been used successfully with people suffering from rheumatoid arthritis, inflammatory bowel disease, asthma, psoriasis, and certain liver diseases. Patients with rheumatoid arthritis are often deficient in folate, and folate stores are decreased in rheumatoid arthritis patients who take methotrexate. Moreover, some of the side effects of the drug, including gastrointestinal distress, mimic folate deficiency. Therefore, patients are often put on high-folate diets or given supplemental folic acid to reduce the side effects with no reduction in the drug's effectiveness. It is recommended that patients with rheumatoid arthritis who are undergoing methotrexate therapy increase folate consumption or supplement with 1,000 micrograms of folic acid per day.

High doses of folate may also interfere with certain anticonvulsant medications used to treat epilepsy, by competing with them for absorption in the intestine. This in turn could interfere with the drugs crossing the barrier to the brain and could lead to seizures.

## Vitamin K

Vitamin K was only discovered about 50 years ago, and like vitamin D, it is made within the human body. Vitamin K is stored in the liver and then distributed throughout the body. It's necessary for the production of proteins found in blood, bones, and kidneys. The AI for vitamin K is 120 micrograms for adult men and 90 micrograms for adult women.

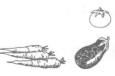

There are at least three different forms of vitamin K, all belonging to a group of chemical compounds called quinones. The naturally occurring, fat-soluble forms are $K_1$ (*phylloquinone*), which occurs in green plants, and $K_2$ (*menaquinone*), which is formed in the intestinal tract in the body as a result of the action of intestinal bacteria. The fat-soluble synthetic vitamin $K_3$ (*menadione*) is nearly twice as potent in the body as the naturally occurring $K_1$ and $K_2$. Vitamin K can be found in a variety of foods, including dried rockweed or dulse seaweed, dried green tea, raw turnip greens, frozen spinach, cooked beef liver, raw cauliflower and broccoli, soybean oil, dried chickpeas and lentils, raw green tomatoes, iceberg lettuce, and strawberries.

## The Benefits of Vitamin K

*Vitamin K and Blood Clotting*

Vitamin K is best known for its important role in blood clotting. At least 13 different proteins are involved in making a blood clot, and vitamin K is essential for the production of at least six of them—especially the protein thrombin. If any of these important proteins are missing, blood cannot clot, which results in hemorrhagic disease. In other words, if an artery or vein is cut the bleeding will not stop.

Hemorrhagic disease is caused by a vitamin K deficiency, which can occur as a result of fat malabsorption (from liver disease, Crohn's disease, or ulcerative colitis) or destruction of the intestinal bacteria by prolonged use of antibiotics. Prior to surgery, patients are sometimes given vitamin K to prevent excess bleeding

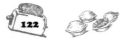

during an operation, but only if a known vitamin K deficiency exists.

*Vitamin K and Bone Health*

Until recently, researchers believed that the body made all of the vitamin K it needed. But new studies indicate that even though the body may make enough vitamin K for blood clotting, it's not necessarily enough for good bone health. In fact, the current RDAs for vitamin K may be too low.

In a 10-year study, part of the Nurses' Health Study at Harvard, researchers looked at the diets of women aged 38 to 63. They found women whose diets contained the most vitamin K (at least 109 micrograms per day) had a 30 percent decreased risk of hip fracture than those who consumed less. This finding supports other data correlating low concentrations of vitamin K in the body with low bone mineral density and bone fractures. This may, in part, be due to the fact that vitamin K is needed to make osteocalcin, the active form of bone protein necessary for bone strength.

## When to Supplement with Vitamin K

Vitamin K deficiency is rare in humans, since we get it through diet and our bodies can make it. However, newborn babies are often susceptible to vitamin K deficiency. Why? First, they're born with a sterile intestinal tract. As they pass through the birth canal they come in contact with the mother's intestinal bacteria, but it often takes the bacteria a day or so to become established in the baby's intestines. Second, babies who are breastfed may not get enough vitamin K, since human milk is a poorer source of the vitamin than infant formula or cow's milk. Infants are at risk of severe cerebral hemorrhage (bleeding in the brain) the first three to four months of life if they do not get enough vitamin K. Therefore, in the United States and in many other countries, newborn babies routinely receive a vitamin K injection at the hospital. People taking sulfa drugs such as the antibiotic Septra may also need extra vitamin K, since these medications can destroy the intestinal bacteria that produce the vitamin. Children, however, do not need vitamin K supplements.

## Niacin

Niacin (pronounced NIGH-uh-sin), or Vitamin B$_3$, was discovered in 1867, but it wasn't until 1937 that scientists realized it was necessary to prevent the disease known as pellagra. Pellagra is characterized by diarrhea, dry/scaly skin, anemia, and eventually, disorientation, memory loss, and confusion. Pellagra is caused by niacin deficiency.

Actually, niacin could be considered the "generic" name for two similar substances: nicotinic acid and niacinamide (or nicotinamide—not related to nicotine found in tobacco). Both nicotinic acid and niacinamide can prevent niacin deficiency. Interestingly, the amino acid tryptophan can also prevent niacin deficiency because the body can convert tryptophan to niacin.

The main function of niacin is as a cofactor for two enzymes that are necessary for the body to convert carbohydrates, proteins, and fats in food into energy. It also helps mobilize calcium from cells and maintains the body's energy supply by controlling how much glucose (bloo sugar) is circulating. Other roles for niacin include keeping skin healthy and helping the digestive and nervous systems function properly.

## The Benefits of Niacin

*Niacin and Heart Disease*

The heart-healthy aspect of niacin stems from its ability to significantly lower blood cholesterol levels, an effect that was first reported in 1955. Nicotinic acid taken in extremely large doses of 1.5 to 3 grams per day has been shown to decrease total cholesterol, LDL ("bad" cholesterol), and triglyceride levels, and increase high-density lipoprotein, or HDL ("good" cholesterol).

ow that this ability to simultane-
HDL and LDL cholesterol in
akes nicotinic acid more effec-
tion cholesterol-lowering drugs
L cholesterol. In fact, the

National Cholesterol Education Program recommends niacin as one of the primary treatments for high cholesterol. Under a doctor's supervision, niacin therapy can also be combined with some prescription cholesterol-lowering drugs for added effectiveness.

### Niacin and Circulatory Disorders

Niacin is known to relax and loosen blood vessels, and therefore may be useful in treating some circulatory disorders such as intermittent claudication, or a limp in one's walk. This disorder is the result of poor circulation and is characterized by painful cramping in the calf that frequently occurs after walking. Raynaud's disease, a disorder in which numbness or pain is experienced in the hands or feet when they're exposed to cold, is another circulatory problem that may be helped by niacin.

*Niacin and Other Potential Benefits*

Although research into additional uses for niacin therapy is preliminary, supplementing with the vitamin may one day prove beneficial for other health problems. For example, people suffering from either rheumatoid arthritis or osteoarthritis may benefit from niacinamide's anti-inflammatory effect. One research study in New Zealand suggests that large doses of niacinamide given to children who are at risk for developing Type 1 diabetes (the insulin-dependent type) may reverse the progression of the disease. And finally, there is limited evidence that niacinamide can ease premenstrual headaches, depression, anxiety, and insomnia. Much more research needs to be completed before niacin is recommended for any of these problems.

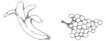

# When to Supplement with Niacin

Most of us get all the niacin we need from the food we eat. Data from the USDA Continuing Survey of Food Intakes by Individuals 1994–96 reveals that the average intake of niacin for Americans is 21.7 milligrams per day—slightly above the current recommended amounts of 16 milligrams niacin equivalents (NE) for adult men and 14 milligrams NE for adult women. Children do not need niacin supplements. Additional survey data indicate that most of our niacin is coming from poultry; mixed dishes that contain a lot of meat, fish, or poultry; enriched and whole-grain breads and bread products; and fortified breakfast cereals.

Niacin is a unique vitamin because, theoretically, it's possible to maintain an adequate

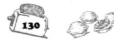  

amount of it in our bodies without eating niacin-containing foods. Why? Because about half of the tryptophan (an amino acid) we eat is converted to niacin. Since tryptophan is found in many common foods, including milk and turkey, a diet containing at least 100 grams of protein could supply us with enough niacin. In fact, when estimating and calculating the required amounts of niacin, the experts took the tryptophan conversion factor into account, which is why the requirements are nearly always expressed in niacin equivalents. A niacin equivalent is equal to 1 milligram of pre-formed niacin or 60 milligrams of tryptophan. Milk and other dairy foods are good sources of niacin because they're high in tryptophan.

*Niacin and Pellagra*

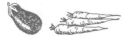 Pellagra (Italian for "raw skin") is a niacin deficiency disease that was first observed in the

mid-eighteenth century in Spain, although at the time the cause wasn't known. In 1920, experts realized that some dietary component lacking in corn was causing pellagra in populations that largely subsisted on corn. It wasn't until 1937 that nicotinic acid was found to be the lacking nutrient.

In scientific experiments with humans, signs of pellagra develop within 50 to 60 days after beginning a niacin-deficient diet. The most common and recognizable signs of a niacin deficiency are changes in the skin. A red rash that looks similar to a sunburn develops in areas exposed to sunlight. Vomiting, constipation, or diarrhea are the classic digestive symptoms of a deficiency, and the tongue becomes bright red. Depression, headache, fatigue, and neurological problems, including loss of memory, also occur.

In the early 1900s, when highly refined cornbread was the main food of poor Americans in the

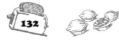

South, asylums were full of patients whose neurological problems were traced to pellagra. Niacin
supplements were the cure, and ultimately corn-
meal was required to be enriched with niacin
(much as the Enrichment Act of 1942 required
food processors to restore the iron, thiamin,
riboflavin, and niacin lost in the milling of wheat).
Although pellagra has now virtually disappeared
from the United States and Europe, it still appears
in India and parts of China and Africa.

There is evidence that niacin deficiency
isn't the only thing that can cause pellagra or
pellagra-like symptoms. Deficiencies of other
nutrients required in the tryptophan-to-niacin
conversion (such as riboflavin, pyridoxine, and
iron) may also be involved in the development
of pellagra. Other conditions, such as the reduction in the conversion of tryptophan to niacin

that occurs with some long-term drug therapies, as well as Hartnup's disease—a genetic disease that affects tryptophan absorption—may also lead to a niacin deficiency. In all of these cases, supplemental niacin brings marked improvements in symptoms, if not an outright cure.

*Niacin and High Cholesterol*

Although extremely effective at bringing down elevated blood cholesterol levels, megadoses of niacin also cause serious side effects. "Niacin flush" is the common name for the red head and neck one gets about 15 to 30 minutes after taking nicotinic acid. The flushing effect can go on for half an hour or longer before wearing off. Other side effects include itching skin, stomach upset, and occasional hyperglycemia (high blood sugar levels).

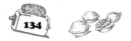

These effects are reversed if the dose of nicotinic acid is reduced or discontinued, and tolerance can be built up by gradually taking larger doses.

Sustained-release, or time-release, nicotinic acid was developed to provide the benefits of niacin without causing niacin flush. It worked well, but unfortunately was later discovered to cause its own set of side effects, including upset stomach, fatigue, and liver damage or liver failure, perhaps due to its chemical structure. Therefore, time-release niacin supplements are no longer recommended. The best way to prevent niacin side effects may be to take the vitamin in the form of inositol hexaniacinate (IHN), available only recently in the United States, although doctors in Europe have prescribed IHN for years. It's just as effective at reducing high cholesterol levels as nicotinic acid, but eliminates the flushing and risk of liver damage. IHN doses higher than 2,000 milligrams per day may also have a blood-thinning effect.

*Niacin and Cardiovascular Risk*

Homocysteine, an amino acid–like substance, has been found to be a risk factor for heart disease when present in high levels in the blood. Results of the Cholesterol Lowering Atherosclerosis Study, published in 1991, showed an increase in blood homocysteine levels in study participants who received niacin and another cholesterol-lowering agent compared with the placebo group. Taking this study one step further to determine if niacin alone would increase homocysteine levels, the year-long Arterial Disease Multiple Intervention Trial was recently conducted with over 450 participants. All participants received 1,000 milligrams of niacin daily for the first four weeks, and an 18 percent increase in average homocysteine levels was noted. Some participants were then assigned to a treatment group and received increasing amounts of niacin—up to 3,000 milligrams per day. The remaining participants received a placebo. In the treatment group homocysteine levels increased a total of 55 percent, while the placebo group experienced declining homocysteine levels. The increase in homocysteine with niacin appeared to be dose related—that is, the more niacin taken, the higher the homocysteine levels.

Although it is not known whether the beneficial effects of niacin on cholesterol levels offset the negative effect it has on homocysteine, the risks of taking large amounts of niacin should be considered when evaluating the usefulness of the vitamin for heart disease patients. One animal study showed that combining niacin and vitamin $B_6$ supplements normalizes homocysteine levels without diminishing the cholesterol-lowering ability of niacin.

## What to Know about Taking Niacin Supplements

- Niacin is sold in tablet and capsule forms. Multivitamins contain about 25 milligrams of niacinamide (or sometimes nicotinic acid); B-complex supplements contain 50 to 100 milligrams of niacinamide; and a single niacin supplement usually contains 500 milligrams.

- Niacin taken in large (and even not-so-large) doses is considered a drug. If you're considering taking niacin in amounts

**138**

greater than those found in multivitamins, talk to your doctor first.

- For circulatory problems, 500 milligrams of IHN is suggested. See your doctor before beginning supplements to make sure this dosage is appropriate for you.

- If, for any reason, you're taking niacin daily for long periods, see your doctor for periodic monitoring of liver function.

- Inadequate iron, riboflavin, or vitamin $B_6$ status decreases the conversion of tryptophan to niacin, but it's currently unknown how much this affects the niacin requirement. Therefore, increasing niacin intake to compensate for this decrease isn't recommended at this time.

- Since dietary supplements (or claims for them) are not reviewed by the Food and Drug Administration, quality control and potency problems may exist with niacin supplements.

# Riboflavin (B$_2$)

Riboflavin (pronounced RIBE-o-flay-vin), also known as vitamin B$_2$, is a yellow, fluorescent compound. Like all B vitamins, riboflavin is water-soluble, but it's more heat-stable than most. Vitamin B$_2$ in the body is found in the form of the coenzymes, flavin mononucleotide (FMN) and flavin-adenine dinucleotide (FAD). FAD, the predominant form of riboflavin, is an essential component of energy production and helps to metabolize carbohydrates, protein, and fat.

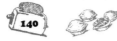

Riboflavin is also involved in the formation of some other vitamins and their coenzymes. FMN, for instance, is required for the conversion of pyridoxine ($B_6$) to its coenzyme, and FAD is required to convert the amino acid tryptophan to niacin.

Although this important nutrient is found in small amounts in the liver and kidneys, it is not stored to any great extent in the body. Therefore, riboflavin must be supplied in the diet and any excess is eliminated through the urine.

## The Benefits of Riboflavin

Preliminary research indicates that taking a high dose of riboflavin (400 milligrams) every day may help prevent migraine headaches. In one study, people who took riboflavin supplements for three months had 37 percent fewer migraines than

**141**

those taking a placebo. Although studies to date have used high doses of riboflavin, further research will investigate the effects of lower doses.

Researchers caution that the riboflavin treatment isn't for everyone. First, you need to make sure that your headaches are true migraines, and second, the treatment is only recommended for people who have migraines at least twice a month.

For those with diagnosed migraines, supplementing with riboflavin might be worth a try. Most riboflavin supplements contain no more than 100 milligrams per tablet, so you'll need a prescription to get one that contains 400 milligrams. Talk to your doctor before treating your migraines with riboflavin supplements.

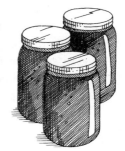

**142**

## Riboflavin in Food

Most plant and animal tissues contain some riboflavin. However, the foods that contribute the most riboflavin to the U.S. diet are milk and milk drinks, followed by bread products and fortified cereals. Riboflavin can also be found in beef liver, yogurt, oranges, baked trout, pork, eggs, fresh cooked spinach, cooked brown rice, and dark meat chicken. National food surveys show that the median daily intake of riboflavin in the United States is about 2 milligrams for men and roughly 1.5 milligrams for women, well above the recommended levels of 1.3 milligrams and 1.1 milligrams, respectively.

## When to Supplement with Riboflavin

Although a true riboflavin deficiency (called ariboflavinosis) is uncommon in the United States, certain groups of people are at a greater risk, including individuals with kidney disease who are being treated with dialysis; individuals with absorption problems; women who are pregnant with more than one fetus; and women who are breast-feeding more than one infant.

Ariboflavinosis can also result from diverse causes, including the use of certain drugs, inadequate dietary intake, rare genetic defects, and hormonal disorders. In addition, chronic diseases such as cancer, heart disease, and diabetes mellitus are known to trigger or exacerbate riboflavin deficiency.

Symptoms of ariboflavinosis include weakness, sore throat, edema (fluid retention) of the mucous membranes in the mouth and throat, cheilosis (dermatitis around the nose and lips), stomatitis

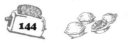

(cracking of the corners of the mouth), photo-phobia (hypersensitivity to light, reddening of cornea), and anemia.

## Thiamin (B₁)

Thiamin (pronounced THIGH-uh-min), also known as vitamin $B_1$, is a water-soluble vitamin. The first B vitamin to be identified, it is found in skeletal muscle, the heart, liver, kidney, and brain.

Thiamin diphosphate (ThDP) is the active form of thiamin and acts as a coenzyme (a small molecule that works with an enzyme to promote the enzyme's activity) in the metabolism of carbohydrate and protein. It is also involved in the synthesis of DNA. As a result, thiamin is also used in a negative way, for tumor growth. In fact, limiting thiamin can slow tumor cell production.

## Thiamin in Food

Although pork and sunflower seeds are the richest sources of thiamin, Americans get most of this vitamin from enriched, fortified, or whole grain products such as bread and bread products, mixed foods whose main ingredient is a grain, and ready-to-eat cereals. Thiamin is also found in baked beans, cooked pasta, and orange juice. The USDA Continuing Survey of Food Intakes by Individuals 1994–96 showed an average intake of 1.9 milligrams of thiamin for males aged 20 and older, and 1.33 milligrams for females aged 20 and older. The recommended intake for thiamin is 1.2 milligrams and

1.1 milligrams per day for adult males and females, respectively.

If you can't get enough of sushi, you might want to think twice. Raw fish contains thiaminase—an enzyme that deactivates thiamin. Cooking fish will make the enzyme inactive.

## When to Supplement with Thiamin

Because the biological half-life of thiamin in the body is about 15 days, deficiency symptoms can be seen in people on a thiamin-deficient diet in as little as 18 days. Although a true thiamin deficiency (called beriberi) is uncommon in the United States, certain groups of people are at a greater risk, including: individuals with kidney disease being treated with dialysis; individuals with malabsorption syndrome or genetic metabolic disorders; women who are pregnant with more than one fetus; seniors; chronic dieters; elite athletes; and alcoholics.

Signs of beriberi primarily involve the nervous and cardiovascular systems and include dementia (mentalconfusion),Wernicke–Korsakoff syndrome (muscle wasting, or "dry" beriberi), edema (wet beriberi), peripheral paralysis, high blood pressure, and an enlarged heart. The "dry" form of beriberi is associated with a low calorie intake and inactivity, with a loss of function or paralysis of the lower limbs. The "wet" form of the deficiency disease, resulting from a high carbohydrate intake and strenuous physical exertion, is associated with edema, or fluid retention, due to heart failure. Beriberi in infants, although rare, is caused by feeding babies thiamin-free formula. The effect can be sudden and rapid, ending in heart failure. Most infant formula in the United States is fortified with thiamin.

In industrialized countries, thiamin deficiency is most often due to a high alcohol intake combined with reduced food consumption. Alcohol can impair the absorption and storage of thiamin, resulting in alcohol-related thiamin deficiency—the third most common form of dementia in the United States.

Treatment of thiamin deficiency often involves 50 to 100 milligram of thiamin/day (given intramuscularly or intravenously) for 7 to 14 days, followed by oral therapy. This treatment can quickly reverse many of the acute symptoms, but often leaves residual neurologic signs such as memory loss (called the chronic phase of Wernicke–Korsakoff syndrome). Recent studies suggest that thiamin deficiency may be related to Alzheimer's disease, although much more research is needed.

# Minerals: Elements of Good Health

## Calcium

Calcium is the most abundant mineral in the human body. Over 99 percent of the body's calcium is found in bones and teeth. The remainder is found in blood, bodily fluids, muscle, and other tissues where it plays a role in blood vessel contraction and dilation, muscle contraction, nerve transmission, and glandular secretion. Calcium is probably most recognized for its important role in maintaining bone health. The skeleton not only provides structural support for muscles, it protects vital organs and serves as a storage site for calcium.

## The Benefits of Calcium

*Calcium and Osteoporosis*

Osteoporosis is a debilitating disease affecting more than 25 million Americans—80 percent of whom are women. Osteoporosis, or porous bone, is caused by low bone mass and the structural deterioration of bone tissue, leading to bone fragility and an increased susceptibility to fractures of the hip, spine, and wrist. Fifty percent of all women over age 50 will have an osteoporosis-related fracture in their lifetime. The incidence of osteoporosis in men is rising. In fact, 20 to 25 percent of all hip fractures in the United States occur in men, and as in women, the chance of occurrence increases dramatically with age. Because of the aging population, the incidence of hip fractures is expected to triple by the year 2040.

In the United States, approximately 21 percent of postmenopausal Caucasian and Asian women, 16 percent of Hispanic women, and 10 percent of African-American women have osteoporosis.

Why are so many women at risk for osteoporosis? A decreased estrogen level beginning at menopause is associated with accelerated bone loss, especially from the lumbar spine, for about five years. During this period a woman may lose an average of 3 percent of her skeletal mass per year! Additionally, lower estrogen levels may decrease calcium absorption and increase rates of bone turnover.

Bone is an active tissue that is constantly undergoing "remodeling" that involves resorption (old bone is removed) and formation (new bone is formed). The rate of remodeling in children can be as high as 50 percent per year compared to about 5 percent in adults. Until the age of 30 or so, we build and store bone efficiently. Then, as part of the aging process, bones begin to break down faster than new bone can be formed. If bone calcium stores are not sufficient, as the aging process takes over, the risk of osteoporosis increases.

Moreover, since bone serves as a "bank" for calcium and other minerals, as blood levels of calcium fall, the mineral is pulled out of the bone via resorption. When blood calcium levels rise, the mineral can be redeposited into the bones in the formation phase. If more calcium is pulled out of the bone than is put into bone,  osteoporosis can occur.

In addition to calcium, magnesium and vitamin D are also needed to prevent osteoporosis. According to experts, calcium increases bone density, but magnesium is involved in the construction of the matrix, a flexible scaffold into which bone tissue is deposited. The matrix allows the skeleton to absorb bone-fracturing shocks. Vitamin D plays an important role in the body's absorption and use of calcium.

*Calcium and Blood Pressure*

In a review of 22 studies, calcium supplementation was found to reduce blood pressure modestly in adults with hypertension, or high blood pressure, but had little effect on people with normal blood pressure. Findings from the recent DASH study (Dietary Approaches to Stop Hypertension) suggest that a diet high in calcium, magnesium, and potassium, and lower in sodium and fat, can lower high blood pressure significantly.

*Calcium and Pre-Eclampsia*

Calcium is now recognized as a treatment for pre-eclampsia, or pregnancy-induced hypertension. In a review of 14 studies, pregnant women who supplemented with 1,500 to 2,000 milligrams of calcium per day had a significant lowering of both their systolic (the top number in a blood pressure reading) and diastolic (the lower number) blood pressure. In another study of 82 pregnant women, those who consumed more than 900 milligrams of calcium (the amount found in three glasses of milk) had lower blood pressure than those who consumed less calcium.

Getting adequate amounts of calcium when pregnant can also save your baby's bones. A

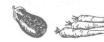

study at the University of Tennessee showed that women who consumed fewer than 600 milligrams of the mineral per day during pregnancy had babies with 15 percent less bone density than babies born to women who consumed up to 2,000 milligrams of calcium per day.

*Calcium and Colon Cancer*

Colon cancer is one of the most common cancers in the Western world. Research has shown that colon cancer incidence rates are inversely proportional to calcium intake—as intakes go up, cancer rates go down. One study indicates that most cases of colon cancer may be prevented with regular calcium intake for men and women around 1,800 milligrams and 1,000 milligrams per 1,000 calories per day, respectively, along with 800 IUs of vitamin D per day.

*Calcium and Premenstrual Syndrome (PMS)*

In a study of 466 premenopausal women, ages 18 to 45, who suffered from recurring premenstrual syndrome (PMS), supplementing with calcium carbonate lessened the symptoms. Researchers gave each woman either 600 milligrams of calcium carbonate or a placebo twice a day for three menstrual cycles. By the third treatment cycle, those taking the calcium supplements reported a 48 percent reduction in overall symptoms during the two weeks prior to their menstrual cycle. Those taking the placebo, however, reported only a 30 percent reduction. The symptoms that improved included depression, mood swings, anxiety, water retention, breast tenderness, cramps, food cravings, and headaches. Insomnia and fatigue did not improve in either group. More

research is needed to determine if other forms
and/or doses of calcium would provide the
same effect.

## Calcium in Food

Calcium is found in a variety of foods,
including dairy products and dark leafy vegetables such as kale, collards, turnip greens, and
broccoli, as well as clams, oysters, and salmon
with bones. According to 1994 data, 73 percent
of the calcium in the U.S. food supply comes
from milk products, 9 percent comes from fruits
and vegetables, 5 percent is from grain products,
and the remaining 12 percent from other
sources. Although grains are not particularly high
in calcium, because they are consumed in such
great quantities, they account for a substantial
proportion of the calcium intake.

## When to Supplement with Calcium

Most Americans do not get the calcium they need. According to a recent statement from the National Institutes of Health, only about 25 percent of boys and 10 percent of girls meet the recommended daily levels of calcium consumption. The USDA Continuing Survey of Food Intakes by Individuals 1994–96 showed an average daily intake of 925 milligrams of calcium for males aged 9 and older, and 657 milligrams for females aged 9 and older. The National Academy of Sciences recently increased the recommended intake of calcium for adults, both male and female, to 1,000 to 1,300 milligrams per day.

Some argue that these new levels are not high enough. Experts at the 1994 NIH Consensus Development Conference on Optimal

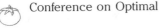

Calcium Intake recommended that women over the age of 50 who are not on estrogen, and all women over the age of 65, should consume 1,500 milligrams of calcium per day. And the American Academy of Pediatrics has recommended that children ages 9 to 18 should also get as much as 1,500 milligrams of calcium per day.

Moreover, certain groups of the population are at greater risk for calcium deficiency, including: menopausal women; young women who lose their periods due to anorexia nervosa and/or exercise-induced anorexia; individuals with lactose intolerance; strict vegetarians; and other individuals with poor calcium intakes. Many chronic illnesses that affect children also affect calcium metabolism and bone formation, including rheumatologic conditions, renal disease, liver failure, and insulin-dependent diabetes mellitus.

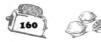

Although lack of calcium is much more common than too much calcium, toxicity can occur with calcium supplementation. Too much calcium can cause kidney stone formation and kidney failure, and it can interfere with the absorption of other nutrients such as zinc, iron, phosphorus, and magnesium.

*Calcium and Other Minerals*

Although calcium and magnesium often work together, they can also compete against one another. Calcium helps muscles contract, while magnesium helps them to relax. However, too much magnesium can inhibit bone hardening, or calcification, while too much calcium can lessen the amount of magnesium absorbed by the body. Therefore, it is essential to maintain a balance between these two minerals. Experts recommend a two-to-one ratio of calcium to magnesium. If you regularly supplement with extra calcium, be sure to increase your magnesium intake, too.

Calcium and iron fight one another for absorption, and calcium can reduce absorption of nonheme iron (the form found in plants, fortified foods, and supplements) when eaten together. On average, though, research has shown that the two nutrients balance out in the long run. For instance, if you eat a bowl of iron-fortified cereal with a cup of milk, you may not absorb all of the iron. On the other hand, vitamin C aids iron absorption, so adding a glass of orange juice can actually increase the amount of iron absorbed from the cereal. The exception is when iron supplements are taken for anemia. In this case, do not take iron supplements at the same time as calcium supplements.

## Choosing a Calcium Supplement

Calcium comes in a variety of forms, including carbonate, citrate, citrate malate, gluconate, phosphate, lactate, and microcrystalline hydroxyapatite. Calcium is also available in fortified foods such as juice, chocolates, yogurt, and cereal. Some calcium sources are better than others, and some are cheaper.

- *Calcium carbonate* is generally the cheapest form of calcium because it's the most concentrated and therefore, fewer supplements are necessary. It should be taken with meals to increase absorption.

- *Calcium citrate malate (CCM)* is available in tablet form and in fortified juice. The low calcium content requires a greater number of tablets per day (2–5 tablets) and it's more expensive. However, studies have

**163**

shown that this particular form of calcium is the best absorbed. Typically, people absorb 35 percent of the calcium in this form, versus 30 percent of the calcium in calcium carbonate and other supplements. The citrate portion may also help reduce the risk of kidney stones.

- *Calcium citrate and calcium lactate* can be taken between meals.
- If you're not a pill-taker, juice fortified with CCM or other calcium forms may be your best bet.


# Chromium

Chromium (pronounced CROW-me-um) is a trace mineral that's essential for maintaining normal blood sugar levels by helping insulin

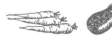

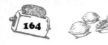   

(a hormone that transfers blood sugar to the body's cells) do its job. It also helps the body break down fats and carbohydrates. There are three forms of chromium used in supplements: chromium picolinate, chromium polynicotinate, and chromium chloride.

## The Benefits of Chromium

*Chromium and Insulin Resistance*

Insulin resistance (sometimes called glucose intolerance) is a condition in which the body's cells don't respond adequately to insulin. Because of this, glucose (blood sugar) doesn't get cleared from the blood as easily, leading to higher circulating blood sugar levels. The pancreas, sensing the need for more insulin, increases its production of the hormone.  Eventually, insulin resistance can lead to diabetes.

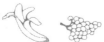

In several studies conducted by the U.S. Department of Agriculture's Beltsville Human Nutrition Research Center, glucose-intolerant people who took 200 micrograms of chromium a day were better able to clear excess glucose from their blood after meals than those who took a placebo. However, the declines in blood sugar levels that were observed, although positive, weren't enough to bring the levels down to normal range. What's more, the results were more striking in those people who consumed a low chromium diet—not those who consumed a normal, varied diet.

In people with insulin resistance, the beneficial effect of chromium supplements is related to the severity of the intolerance. That is, chromium

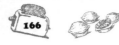

only seems to work for people who are insulin resistant; people with good glucose tolerance do not respond to supplemental chromium.

*Chromium and Diabetes*

People with diabetes have a higher requirement for chromium since they have impaired mechanisms to convert chromium to a usable form in the body. Although 200 micrograms might be helpful with glucose intolerance, it isn't enough to produce a positive effect with Type 2 diabetes.

A number of research studies with diabetics have yielded positive results with chromium supplements of 400 to 1,000 micrograms per day. In these people, insulin sensitivity and action was increased, and blood sugar control was better. And, although chromium picolinate appeared to be more effective than chromium chloride supplements in some studies, this has not been shown across the board. Diabetics should discuss chromium supplementation with their doctors.

*Chromium and Other Potential Benefits*

Two of the most popular claims made for chromium supplements—and the ones that probably lure the most consumers to the supplements—are that chromium picolinate causes fat loss and weight loss, and that it increases muscle mass. In truth, these claims are largely unsupported. Only a few small studies were conducted—all by one researcher—and he used a scientifically unreliable measuring tool (testing body fat

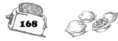   
levels with calipers). Follow-up studies using a more reliable measurement of fat and muscle (underwater weighing) have shown no effect of chromium supplementation on muscle, fat, or weight. In fact, in November of 1996, the Federal Trade Commission ordered one chromium picolinate supplement manufacturer to stop making unsubstantiated weight loss and health claims for their supplement.

## When to Supplement with Chromium

Although there's no RDA for chromium (it's unknown exactly how much the body needs), it's widely agreed that most people probably don't get enough from their diets. Some estimates put typical consumption between 25 and 35 micrograms per day—short of the Adequate Intake level for some groups.

The AI for men between the ages of 14 and 50 is 35 micrograms. For women between 19 and 50, the AI is 25 micrograms. After age 50, the AI goes down to 30 micrograms for men and 20 micrograms for women. For most people, a varied diet along with a chromium-containing multivitamin should be sufficient. Children should not take chromium supplements.

Although side effects from chromium appear to be rare, there have been some reports of skin reactions from chromium picolinate supplements. It's also possible that chromium supplements will induce anemia in women who take them for more than a few months.

A recent research report linking chromium picolinate supplements to cancer in animals garnered plenty of media attention. Apparently, the picolinate part of the supplement is the problem—

**170**

not the chromium part. Of course, negative findings such as this are always cause for some concern. However, this was only one study, and therefore its conclusions should not be accepted as a final answer on chromium safety (just as one study on a chromium benefit shouldn't be accepted as the whole story). If you're determined to use a chromium supplement, don't choose one with picolinate. Or, use supplemental brewer's yeast, which has chromium but no picolinate.

## Iron

The most studied and best understood mineral, iron was identified as a component of blood back in the eighteenth century. About three-fourths of the body's iron is found in hemoglobin, a key component of red blood cells. Hemoglobin's job is to deliver oxygen to the body's cells and carry carbon dioxide—a waste product—away from the cells to the lungs. Exhaling rids the body of the carbon dioxide. The rest of the body's iron is found in enzymes and myoglobin (temporary iron storage in the muscles and heart) with longer-term storage in the liver, spleen, and bone marrow. Iron can be found in a variety of foods, including clams, beef liver, ground beef, chicken legs, canned beans and franks, fortified cereals, enriched white rice, cashews, whole wheat bread, eggs, and milk.

## The Benefits of Iron

*Iron and Anemia*

Iron deficiency anemia is characterized by low iron stores and depressed hemoglobin production. Anemia decreases the amount of

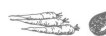

oxygen delivered to the body tissues. The body compensates for this by extracting more oxygen from hemoglobin, redistributing blood flow to vital organs at the expense of other tissues, and making the heart work harder to circulate the blood. These compensatory measures put stress on the body, and when combined with other disease states or medical problems, extreme illness can result.

Symptoms of anemia come on gradually and include pale skin, weakness, lack of energy, breathlessness, inability to maintain body temperature, increased susceptibility to infections, and irregular heartbeat. During pregnancy, anemia increases the risk of having a premature and low birth weight baby. In young children, iron deficiency is associated with learning disabilities and behavioral problems such as reduced attention span, as well as increased absorption of lead. In fact, in the United States, children who have iron deficiency have a three to four times higher prevalence of lead poisoning than children who aren't iron deficient.

Iron supplementation is highly effective at reversing anemia, producing results after about one month of treatment. (If there is no correction after a month, further medical evaluation is necessary—there may be other causes for the anemia.) In children, research in many countries shows that iron therapy can help reverse the learning problems associated with anemia, but it may not be 100 percent effective in this regard. Some studies suggest that children who experienced iron deficiency at a young age and over a long time never catch up to their peers intellectually.

## When to Supplement with Iron

In the United States, where meat consumption is generally high, most people have little difficulty meeting the Recommended Dietary Allowance for iron—the exception to this is girls and women who are menstruating. The USDA Continuing Survey of Food Intakes by Individuals in 1996 revealed that the average iron intake for females aged 20 and over was 13 milligrams; for males it was 19 milligrams. The RDA for iron is 11 milligrams for males ages 14 to 18 and 8 milligrams for men 19 and older. For women ages 14 to 18 years, the RDA is 15 milligrams. For women ages 19 to 50 years old, the RDA is 18 milligrams, and for women 51 and older, the RDA is 8 milligrams. Only supplement children with iron if prescribed by a physician.

*Iron Deficiency*

Iron deficiency is the most common nutritional deficiency in the United States and worldwide, affecting mainly older infants, young children, and females of childbearing age. In developing countries it's estimated that 30 to 40 percent of young children and premenopausal women are deficient in iron. In the United States, the third National Health and Nutrition Examination Survey, conducted in 1991, showed that about 5 percent of children aged 1 to 2 had iron deficiency, and about half of those were anemic as well.

Iron deficiency most commonly occurs as a result of increased needs during periods of growth—pregnancy, infancy, early childhood, and puberty, for example. Breastfed infants can be at risk if they aren't receiving supplemental

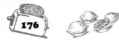

iron or aren't eating iron-fortified foods. Women in the childbearing years require about twice the iron of men in order to cover menstrual blood losses. Adolescent females are particularly at risk for deficiency because they're growing *and* they're losing blood. Individuals who have suffered blood loss (i.e., from an accident) are also at risk for iron deficiency.

A person who is iron deficient isn't automatically anemic; iron deficiency progresses in three stages. First, iron stores in the bone marrow, liver, and spleen are depleted. Next, red blood cell production is reduced, and finally, hemoglobin production falls, resulting in anemia. Blood tests can diagnose iron deficiency in any of these stages.

The body has an interesting way to fight against iron deficiency. As is the case with many nutrients, when the body is low on iron, it adapts to absorb more. However, the body goes one step further in the case of iron. Studies show that when the diet is high in nonheme iron (from plant foods) but contains little heme iron (from animal products), the body increases its ability to absorb nonheme iron. This enables people who derive their iron primarily from vegetable sources to better maintain their body stores. The diet does not need to contain animal products for proper iron intake. Iron is also contained in iron-fortified products such as cereals and breads, so vegetarians don't have to consume animal products. (This adaptation does not appear to work in reverse. In other words, the body does not begin to absorb less iron when a high heme iron diet is consumed.)

Iron deficiency is effectively treated with iron supplements, which have been used since 1832.

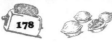

They efficiently reverse iron deficiency and can correct iron-deficiency anemia. However, they frequently produce gastrointestinal side effects, the most common of which are nausea and constipation. The risk of side effects is directly proportional to the iron dose. According to experts, doses larger than 120 milligrams are the most likely to cause unpleasant symptoms. Such large doses are not necessary in most cases.

*WARNING: Children and Iron Poisoning*
According to the Food and Drug Administration, iron-containing supplements are the leading cause of pediatric poisoning deaths for children under age six in the United States. Between June 1992 and January 1993, five toddlers died after eating iron supplements,

according to the national Centers for Disease Control and Prevention.

Iron poisoning in children causes problems within minutes or hours after ingestion. Early symptoms include nausea, vomiting, diarrhea, and gastrointestinal bleeding, developing into shock, coma, seizures, and death. Even if no symptoms appear, or if the child seems to be recovering, medical treatment is necessary. A child who survives iron poisoning can experience health problems (gastrointestinal obstruction and liver damage) up to a month after the incident.

Iron supplements are tempting to children because they frequently look like candy. They're round and often red in color, and some have a sweet-tasting coating to cover up the bad-tasting iron. In 1993, the Nonprescription Drug Manufacturers Association, which includes companies that manufacture about 95 percent of the nonprescription medicines available today, adopted a policy that called for the elimination of sweet coatings on iron-containing supplements that provided 30 milligrams or more iron per dose. They also agreed to new voluntary warning labels for these products. In 1997, FDA required "unit-dose" packaging for iron-containing products with 30 milligrams or more of iron per dose. This packaging features individual "bubbles" from which a paper or foil covering must be peeled before the supplement will come out. It's believed that this packaging will discourage children from taking the supplements, or at least limit the number of tablets a child would swallow. This requirement is in addition to existing U.S. Consumer Product Safety Commission regulations, which

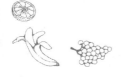

require child-resistant packaging for most iron-containing products.

If you suspect a child has overdosed on an iron-containing supplement, call the nearest poison control center or the child's physician first, then follow their instructions. Of course, taking steps to avoid an iron-poisoning situation first is the best plan.

*Hemochromatosis*

Overloading the body's iron stores by chronically taking too much supplemental iron (or sometimes by blood transfusions) can damage various organs by causing excessive iron storage. The best known, and probably the most common, form of chronic iron overload is hereditary hemochromatosis. Of course, people diagnosed with the disease should not take iron supplements.

In population groups with European ancestry, approximately three in 1,000 have hemochromatosis, a genetic abnormality that causes a greater than normal absorption of iron. The organs most affected are the liver, heart, pancreas, and pituitary gland; the joints are also impacted. When total body iron accumulates to 20 to 40 grams (about 10 percent more than normal), signs of the abnormality—including arthritis, diabetes, cirrhosis of the liver, sexual dysfunction, and heart failure—begin to show. Although it can vary, symptoms of hemochromatosis don't usually surface until later in life, when bodily needs for iron have decreased—that's why many people with this disorder don't even know they have it. In men symptoms typically appear around age 30 to 50; in women, it's after menopause.

183

Even if you have no symptoms, it's not difficult to be screened for hemochromatosis. A simple blood test will reveal if your transferrin (protein in the blood that carries iron) is saturated with iron. The main treatment for the disease is phlebotomy, or removal of blood from the body. When phlebotomy is started before clinical signs of the disease appear, organ damage can be prevented. However, the treatment will not reverse organ damage that has already occurred. For this reason, screening is recommended for people who may be at risk for hemochromatosis—even if they show no symptoms.

Some research has linked high iron levels with cancer, increased rates of tumor growth, and coronary heart disease. With the exception of an increased risk of liver cancer among people with hemochromatosis (due to chronic injury of the

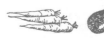

liver from high levels of iron stored there), further study has not supported these associations.

## Zinc

Although zinc has been known to be an essential mineral for more than 50 years, for much of that time it was considered a relatively unimportant nutrient. However, the past few years have seen interest in zinc increase dramatically—not only in nutrition and health circles, but among consumers as well. Why the sudden interest? Numerous new studies about zinc's many functions show it to be of crucial importance to human health. Zinc is a component of more than 200 enzymes, which are necessary for many bodily processes. Zinc is also essential for growth,

immune system function, taste and smell sensation,
reproductive health, wound healing, and more.

## The Benefits of Zinc

*Zinc and Immunity*

Even moderate degrees of zinc deficiency can
compromise the immune system. T-cell lymphocytes, the white blood cells that help fight infection,
don't function well when zinc stores are low.
Therefore, people who are zinc-deficient have a
more difficult time resisting infections. Research
has shown that when zinc supplements are given
to individuals with low zinc levels, the numbers of
T-cell lymphocytes circulating in the blood
increase, and the ability of these cells to fight infection improves. Limited data also suggest that the
incidence of certain respiratory infections and
malaria may also be reduced by zinc supplements.

*Zinc and the Common Cold*

There is much debate about whether zinc lozenges help make colds more bearable. A study of more than 100 employees of the Cleveland Clinic suggested that sucking on zinc lozenges decreased the duration of colds by one-half—or about three days—and lessened the severity of colds as well. This study has been criticized by some researchers, since zinc lozenges are known for their unappealing taste—a factor that could make it obvious to study participants whether they were taking the zinc or the placebo lozenges, thereby skewing the study results. Other studies have found no effect from zinc lozenges.

It's important to note that the lozenges used in these studies contained zinc gluconate. Other forms of zinc, such as zinc acetate, zinc aspartate, and zinc citrate, which are found in some "cold season" products, have *no* published studies to back up their claims for alleviating cold symptoms.

If you decide to take zinc gluconate lozenges for a cold, begin taking them every few hours as soon as your symptoms show up. Don't exceed the recommended dosage, and don't take the lozenges for more than a week. Taking zinc supplements (tablets, capsules, etc.) won't work for colds because the form used to make the lozenges, zinc gluconate, is generally not available in capsule form. This is the best form for treating colds.

*Zinc and Wound Healing*

Zinc supplements have been shown to increase rates of wound healing, including burns. Skin irritations and bedsores are helped by zinc supplements (not lozenges), but only if the person is zinc-deficient in the first place. In other words, when zinc levels are normal, taking zinc supplements to help a wound heal doesn't work.

*Zinc and Other Potential Benefits*

There are many other purported benefits of zinc supplements, but the scientific research to support such uses of the mineral is preliminary, contradictory, or significantly lacking at this time. Some of these uses for zinc include the treatment of rheumatoid arthritis and lupus, which involve the immune system. Zinc is necessary to make testosterone and other hormones, so it may be useful for enhancing fertility in both women and men. Zinc may also slow vision loss in people with macular degeneration, a common cause of blindness in those over age 50. Osteoporosis, hemorrhoids, inflammatory bowel disease, prostatic hypertrophy (enlarged prostate gland), and ulcers are other health problems for which zinc may eventually prove beneficial.

## Zinc in Food

Zinc is found in protein foods. Beef, pork, organ meats, poultry (especially dark meat), eggs, and seafood (especially oysters) are the best sources. Other sources include beans, nuts, seeds, and wheat germ. According to experts, people eating a typical Western diet get about half of their dietary zinc from meat, fish, and poultry. Another 20 percent comes from dairy products, some comes from grains, and a small amount from beans, nuts, and soy products.

Humans absorb only about 33 percent of the total zinc in our diets. Zinc from animal foods is better absorbed than zinc from plant foods (because of the fiber and phytic acid contained in plants). This can be a problem for strict vegetarians or vegans whose diets contain lots of high-fiber foods. Also, infants absorb less zinc when fed soy-based formula, which contains phytate, than when fed a milk-based formula.

## When to Supplement with Zinc

The RDA for zinc is 11 milligrams for adult men and pregnant women 19 or older. For adult women, the RDA is 8 milligrams. Extra zinc is needed during periods of rapid growth, pregnancy, and lactation. However, according to two national surveys, the National Health and Nutrition Examination Survey (1988–91) and the USDA Continuing Survey of Food Intakes of Individuals 1994–96, pregnant and breastfeeding women (as well as people aged 51 and older) don't get the recommended amounts of zinc. Additional surveys also revealed that young children, aged one to six years, adolescents, and low-income adults also consume less than the recommended amounts. However, consult your pediatrician before giving children zinc supplements.

The body works hard to maintain the proper level of zinc by increasing its absorption efficiency

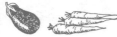

The earliest sign of zinc deficiency is poor appetite, followed by weight loss, taste abnormalities, mental lethargy, and slow healing of wounds. With chronic, severe zinc deficiency, these symptoms worsen and are joined by hair loss, diarrhea, skin rashes, depressed immune function and increased susceptibility to infections, delayed fetal development and reduced growth (in children and adolescents), impaired vision, and reproductive dysfunction.

Large doses of zinc (150 milligrams and greater) have been shown to cause nausea, vomiting, and dizziness. Over time, zinc intakes of 150 to 450 milligrams per day result in reduced immune function and reduced levels of HDL ("good" cholesterol) as well. The National Academy of Sciences is currently evaluating the long-term risk of taking zinc supplements.